Coping with Birth Trauma and Postnatal Depression

D1635060

Overcoming Common Problems Series

Selected titles

Overcoming Common Problems Series

Overcoming Common Problems Series

Overcoming Common Problems Series

Coping with Birth Trauma and Postnatal Depression

LUCY JOLIN

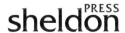

First published in the UK in 2008 by the Sheldon Press

This revised and updated edition published 2019 by Sheldon Press
An imprint of John Murray Press
An Hachette UK company

1

British Library Cataloguing-in-Publication Data

A catalogue record for this book is available from the British Library.

Trade Paperback ISBN 978 1 52932 9 155
eBook ISBN 978 1 52938 5 618

Every reasonable effort has been made to trace copyright holders, but if there
are any errors or omissions, Nicholas Brealey will be pleased to insert the ap-
propriate acknowledgement in any subsequent printings or editions.

Typeset by Cenveo® Publisher Services.
Printed and bound in Great Britain by Clays Ltd, Elcograf S.p.A.

John Murray Press policy is to use papers that are natural, renewable and
recyclable products and made from wood grown in sustainable forests.
The logging and manufacturing processes are expected to conform to the
environmental regulations of the country of origin.

Sheldon Press
Carmelite House
50 Victoria Embankment
London EC4Y 0DZ

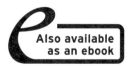

Also available
as an ebook

To Dan, Louis and Max
I couldn't have done it without you

Contents

About the author

Lucy Jolin is a freelance journalist who has written for numerous national magazines, newspaper and websites on a wide range of subjects, ranging from birth trauma to the power of play. She is married to Dan and has two sons, Louis and Max.

Foreword

Many years ago my friend Stella had a baby. She was in her late twenties, strong and healthy – a good candidate for a straightforward birth. But when I visited her in hospital a few days after her baby was born, she immediately, and uncharacteristically, burst into tears. Telling me the story of her birth, she explained that she had been left to labour in pain for more than 30 hours. When staff realised that the baby wasn't going to arrive on its own, Stella was given a general anaesthetic and her baby girl was born by forceps. She weighed just under 4.5 kilos (10 pounds).

Over the months that followed, I saw Stella a few times, and knew that something wasn't right. She kept returning to the subject of the birth and what had gone wrong. At the time, I didn't know how to help – none of my other friends had had babies.

When we both moved away to different places, we lost touch, but I thought of her frequently, particularly when other friends started to have children and my own daughter was born. It eventually occurred to me that she almost certainly had undiagnosed postnatal depression (PND), and that, later still, she probably had post-traumatic stress disorder (PTSD) as well. In the 1980s maternal mental health was something that was poorly understood, even by professionals.

It was partly because of Stella that I became interested in how women's mental health is affected by childbirth and motherhood. Since I became involved with the Birth Trauma Association, a charity that supports women with postnatal PTSD, I've heard many, many stories like Stella's: from women who had long, difficult labours, or who experienced birth injuries, or who didn't see their babies until hours after they'd been born. Many relive their experience several times a day, through flashbacks and nightmares, and are constantly on high alert for signs of danger. Feelings of intense fear and dread can be triggered by something as simple as walking past a hospital or hearing another woman's birth story.

One of the hardest things about becoming a mother is that, at the point when we are most in need of rest and recuperation, we are thrown into a world of sleepless nights and full-time care for another human being, with little time to look after ourselves. So it's not surprising that some women find the experience of early motherhood very different from what they'd hoped and imagined. They are unable to bond with their baby, and the exhaustion, drudgery and sheer loneliness of looking after a newborn leave them feeling depressed and despairing.

As if that wasn't enough, we find that, instead of sympathy, new mothers often attract judgement: for breastfeeding, or not breastfeeding; for co-sleeping, or for putting baby in a cot; for using sleep-training techniques, or for picking up our baby as soon as it cries. No wonder so many of us feel plagued by guilt.

A couple of years ago Stella and I got back in touch. After we'd chatted a little while, we talked again about her birth experience, and I realized that, even 25 years later, it was still vivid in her mind. Sadly, this isn't uncommon: at the Birth Trauma Association, we've learned that the impact of a traumatic birth can be profound and long-lasting. Although the medical profession now has a much better understanding of the mental health problems women can face after childbirth and how to treat them, there is so much more that could be done. Women are still sometimes told to snap out of it, or admonished to be thankful that they've got a healthy baby. If only it were that easy.

This book is one I wish I could have given my friend all those years ago. Lucy Jolin has written a completely non-judgemental guide to postnatal depression and birth trauma. Having been through these experiences herself, she understands the emotional distress so many women go through, and how lonely they can feel. Her book is packed with good advice about learning to love your baby, negotiating relationships with your family and looking after your own needs. The biggest takeaway is that you are not alone: it's not unusual to feel like this, and there is light at the end of the tunnel.

If you are a mother who feels traumatized or depressed, and that you have nowhere to turn, then take heart: you have done the right thing by picking up this book. Read this wise, compassionate and thoughtful guide to coping with birth trauma and postnatal depression, and know that you are taking the first step to recovery.

Dr Kim Thomas, CEO, The Birth Trauma Association

Introduction

This is not a book about how horrible it is to be a mother. There are few sensations more memorable than holding your child close, breathing in his special smell, seeing him toddle away from you across the kitchen for the first time with that funny baby-animal walk, or observing his delighted face when he sees a giraffe for the first time. Children are wonderful. That's why we have them.

But what's so hard to come to terms with – and to explain to others – are the negative feelings that make up the flip side, the difficult aspects of motherhood. The health visitor has signed you off, your partner is back at work, the last bunch of flowers has been consigned to the compost and now you're on your own. When you're bruised and exhausted from the birth and faced with a screaming baby at four in the morning on a freezing January night, it seems impossible that life will ever get better. You can't imagine an end to those long, lonely days when all you ever seem to do is feed, change nappies and stare at the wall.

I certainly found the transition to motherhood hard. I had dreamed of a natural birth for my son. In the event, I went into labour a month early and wasn't allowed to go to the birth centre, with its big pools and partner-friendly policies. I ended up as I'd always feared, flat on my back and attached to about six different catheters, monitors and drips.

My son was born after a gruelling 20-hour labour. The cord was round his neck twice. It kept dragging him back inside me, which is why the doctor had to eventually pull him out with forceps. When the midwife put him on my breast, I felt nothing. The hospital insisted on keeping us in for three days. When we finally got home, I burst into tears. I remember telling my husband: 'Now I've got him home, I don't know what to do with him.' The next day the midwife came round, told us my son was severely jaundiced and that we should take him straight back to hospital. We stayed there for another four days, during which time I seriously considered walking out of the hospital and up the dual carriageway until I collapsed. I often wonder whether

I should have run away. Perhaps help would have been more forthcoming if I had.

Back home again, I felt terrified and utterly alone. My family were wonderful but I was too afraid to ask for more help. I cried every day for four months. I was too scared to tell my health visitor how I felt.

Before the birth, I had been a happy and confident woman, eagerly looking forward to what I was sure would be a little bundle of joy. Now I felt like a robot, mechanically cleaning and feeding my son but feeling nothing for him. I was afraid to go to mother and baby groups in case they were filled with joyful, fulfilled mums. Everywhere I looked, other women seemed to be having a wonderful time – why wasn't I?

Everything changes after having a baby, in ways you can't imagine. We're all as prepared as we can be for the practical aspects – nappy changing, breastfeeding, disturbed nights and so on. But how do you cope with the negative emotions? When you burst into tears every time you relive your baby's birth? When seeing a positive birth story on a Facebook or an Instagram post sends you into a spiral of depression? When you don't feel the love and fulfilment that every other woman seems to feel? And when your partner, who before the birth seemed tuned in to your every emotion, now battles to understand what you're going through?

Of course, not everyone feels like this. Many women find that motherhood fulfils them in a way they never thought possible. The birth itself may not have been the greatest experience of their lives, but they are able to move on. They bond with their child. And they may find it hard to understand that other women don't feel the same.

How many of us find motherhood hard? In terms of bald statistics, experts estimate that one in six new mothers will suffer from postnatal depression. Some believe that the real figure is much higher, since many women find it hard to admit that they are feeling depressed. The Birth Trauma Association estimates that up to 200,000 women each year may feel traumatized by childbirth. Around 30,000 develop PTSD as a result. There are certainly a lot of unhappy new mothers out there.

We have high expectations of motherhood. This is hardly surprising: after all, a flourishing industry has sprung up around it. With soft-focus images, calming music and reassuring words, they promise us a picture-perfect birth and early motherhood experience: everything will be fine if we read the right books, do the right exercises, follow the right Instagram accounts, buy the right buggy or blanket. So we do what we are told to do, and then we are told that we were stupid to believe it would help. Debates over whether women's 'high expectations' of birth contribute to our negative feelings afterwards are commonplace. There is a name for that kind of unpleasantness: victim-blaming.

When I wrote the first edition of this book, talking about birth trauma and postnatal depression was a taboo subject. It was rare to find women who were prepared to go public with how they felt. When I decided to write about my experiences of both, in one of the UK's biggest-selling women's magazines, I was astonished at the large and positive response, but perhaps I shouldn't have been. I thought I was a freak. In fact, I was normal. Since then, the public profile of birth trauma and postnatal depression has rocketed. On the one hand, I'm delighted to see that so many women now feel able to share their stories and seek support: the Birth Trauma Association's peer-to-peer support page on Facebook now has more than 7,000 members. On the other, I'm sad that this rise in awareness hasn't necessarily led to a rise in the help available to us.

This book discusses those aspects of motherhood that the celebrities don't seem so keen to share with their adoring public. It covers birth trauma, postnatal depression, changing relationships with loved ones, bonding with your baby, finding your own parenting style, and learning to live with your new life and body shape. Everyone has his or her own opinions about parenthood, and I will not be forcing mine on you. I'll just be helping you find the path that suits you and your family best.

I would like to thank the wonderful women who talked to me for this book. Some of them are friends and colleagues, but most responded to requests for help on Mumsnet and Netmums forums. These women, none of whom had ever met or spoken to me before, willingly gave up their precious time to talk to me about painful, traumatic or humiliating experiences. None of them is fully identified in the book, because I wanted them to be able to talk without fear of reprisals. Ladies, you know who you are and I can't thank you enough. I would also like to thank the Birth Trauma Association, where I spent several very happy years as a volunteer media officer and was privileged to hear the stories and experiences of many mothers who helped us carry on raising awareness of the condition.

It has been a long, strange road to joyful motherhood for me, and I would have liked to have had a book to help me along the way. There are thousands of books, courses and websites aimed at helping you to have the perfect birth. Most end at the hospital doors. But once the pain relief wears off, that is when you need help, reassurance and support the most. And it helps to know you're not alone.

1
Coming to terms with a traumatic birth

Four themes emerged that described the essence of women's experiences of birth trauma: To care for me: Was that too much to ask? To communicate with me: Why was this neglected? To provide safe care: You betrayed my trust and I felt powerless, and: The end justifies the means: At whose expense? At what price?

Cheryl Beck, Professor of Nursing, University of Connecticut

Throughout my pregnancy, I never heard anyone mention birth trauma. My own mother had five children, with no pain relief for any except the first (and that was given to her against her will). So I always assumed I'd be fine.

After the birth of my son, I couldn't understand why I was unable to stop obsessing about it. In fact, my worries about whether having an epidural was 'the right thing to do' started while I was having it. For months afterwards, I was still beating myself up. I'd have terrible dreams in which I was pinned down on a bed, unable to escape. Every time I thought about my labour, I cried but I couldn't really say why – after all, I was OK, wasn't I? I hadn't died, my baby hadn't died; I should be grateful and stop moaning.

It is possible to recover from birth trauma, but, in order to recover from it you first have to recognize it and admit it. It's not a widely known condition. It's not something your midwife is likely to ask about, and it's not something your friends are likely to admit to. If you think you are suffering from birth trauma, well done; you have taken the first step to recovery.

Cath
I feel as if I've been lied to by every mother I know (how come they all say they feel the things that I've never felt?). The birth (although a straightforward seven hours) absolutely terrified me too – it wasn't nature at its greatest as far as I was concerned. And as for when my daughter was born, there were gasps and tears of joy from everyone except me. I just lay there with the baby on my chest, wondering what the hell I was supposed to feel next.

What is birth trauma?

It's useful to define what we mean by birth trauma, since the term is also used by medical professionals to describe physical injuries sustained by a mother or child during birth. The Birth Trauma Association defines the kind we're discussing here as PTSD following birth, so that's how I'll refer to it here from now on.

Though most of us are familiar with the concept of PTSD following, for example, a hugely traumatic event, such as a rape, a terrorist attack or a car accident, it's sometimes hard to believe that it can be connected with a 'natural' event like birth. In particular, it can be difficult to come to terms with the fact that an event that is commonly supposed to be the happiest of a woman's life can cause PTSD.

However, an increasing body of evidence suggests that PTSD can indeed follow childbirth. As the Birth Trauma Association points out:

> A traumatic experience can be any experience involving the threat of death or serious injury to an individual or another person close to them (e.g. their baby) so it is now understood that PTSD can be a consequence of a traumatic birth.

The very existence of PTSD following childbirth has been questioned. It was posited by the American Psychiatric Association in its *Diagnostic and Statistical Manual of Mental Disorders* (DSM III) that PTSD can occur only after a stressful, abnormal event. Childbirth, it reasoned, falls within our common experience and therefore cannot be seen as 'abnormal'. However, a later edition published in 2000 (DSM-IV-TR) widened the definition of a stressful event to one seen as threatening by a victim or a witness. Childbirth would certainly fall into this category.

The most recent edition (DSM-5), published in 2013, defines the trigger to PTSD as exposure to actual or threatened death, serious injury or sexual violation. The exposure must result from one or more of the following scenarios, in which the individual:

- directly experiences the traumatic event;
- witnesses the traumatic event in person;

- learns that the traumatic event occurred to a close family member or close friend (with the actual or threatened death being either violent or accidental);
- experiences first-hand repeated or extreme exposure to aversive details of the traumatic event (not through media, pictures, television or movies unless work-related).

It could also be argued that, particularly in the case of a first birth, most women living in the developed world will never have seen another woman giving birth, and therefore the experience is very far from normal. My experience of birth was limited to a video in biology class at the age of 15 (my main memories of the lesson are of a general chorus of 'yucks' and 'ughs', with one girl running out of the class claiming she was going to be sick) and numerous TV births, which seemed to consist mostly of blood-spattered delivery rooms, yelling doctors and screaming mothers. These unfortunates usually either died, leaving their weeping husbands cradling the suddenly blood-and-mucus-free infant, or had miraculous escapes and were happily drinking tea with not a hair out of place five minutes later. I suspect that many women of my generation had exactly the same experience as me, with absolutely no idea of the realities of birth until we found ourselves in the stirrups.

The incidence of PTSD following childbirth is now generally accepted to be around 2–5 per cent. However, several studies have found higher incidences. Soet, Brack and Delorio identified PTSD in 34 per cent of participants, with 1.9 per cent developing all the symptoms of PTSD and 30.1 per cent developing some symptoms. Czarnocka and Slade found that 3 per cent of subjects showed 'clinically significant levels' of PTSD and 24 per cent showed some symptoms – and this was in a study of women who had had 'normal' births. Creedy, Shochet and Horsfall found that one in three women interviewed had at least three trauma symptoms, while a further 5.6 per cent met the criteria for acute PTSD. It's also important to note that PTSD following childbirth is not just a problem for mothers in the developed world. Adewuya, Ologu and Ibigbami's study of PTSD following childbirth among Nigerian women found a 5.9 per cent incidence.

On a purely anecdotal level, not one of the women I interviewed for this chapter had sought any medical advice for her PTSD, suggesting that the unreported numbers could be far higher. Most felt that they should 'get over it' by themselves, while others were worried about having a psychiatric disorder on their medical records.

Jane
I'm from a family of copers. So I coped.

A brief history of birth

Birth trauma is presumably as old as birth. Until recently, women could rely on little except luck once they went into labour (and this is still the case in many parts of the world). If you were rich, you could use an experienced doctor or favoured midwife. If you were poor, the best you could expect was the local wise woman or your mother. Deaths of mothers and babies were commonplace. Pain was a given.

In fact, when pain relief was first introduced, many doctors questioned its use for birth. Women should feel pain, they argued. It was a necessary part of childbirth, laid down by God himself following, in biblical tradition, Eve's transgression in the Garden of Eden: 'Unto the woman he said, I will greatly multiply thy sorrow and thy conception; in sorrow thou shalt bring forth children' (Genesis 3.16).

In 1853, pain relief during childbirth took a huge step forward when Dr John Snow administered chloroform to Queen Victoria during the birth of her son, Prince Leopold. As he was her eighth child, it's hardly surprising that Victoria was eager to try out new methods of pain relief. However, this radical new treatment was scorned by the medical journal *The Lancet*, which pontificated in an editorial:

> In no case could it be justifiable to administer chloroform in perfectly ordinary labour; but the responsibility of advocating such a proceeding in the case of the Sovereign of these realms would, indeed, be tremendous. Probably some officious meddlers about the Court so far overruled Her Majesty's responsible

professional advisers as to lead to the pretence of administering chloroform, but we believe the obstetric physicians to whose ability the safety of our illustrious Queen is confided do not sanction the use of chloroform in natural labour.

Snow himself reported:

> I commenced to give a little chloroform with each pain, by pouring about 15 minims by measure on a folded handkerchief. The first stage of labour was nearly over when the chloroform commenced. Her Majesty expressed great relief from the application, the pains being trifling during the uterine contractions, and whilst between the periods of contraction there was complete ease.

Following the successful delivery, 'the Queen appeared very cheerful and well, expressing herself much gratified with the effect of the chloroform'.

The respectable doctors of *The Lancet* might have disapproved, but the Queen's example meant pain relief was here to stay. Doctors and hospital births gradually became the norm, while the number of home births attended solely by midwives dropped. Chloroform gradually gave way to heavy-duty drugs such as morphine and scopolamine. Maternity care moved from bedrooms to labour wards.

However, the medicalization of birth brought new problems for labouring women to cope with. The use of heavy straps and stirrups to keep drugged women under control, and enemas to 'clean them out' before birth, became commonplace. My mother recalls doctors cheerily catheterizing her without anaesthetic just moments after the birth of my brother in the 1970s, as part of a 'study'. 'That pain was worse than the birth,' she told me.

As soon as they were born, it was common practice to remove babies from their mothers, give them a good scrub and put them in separate wards, to be brought to their mothers at specified feeding times. As early as 1958, US magazines were describing 'horrors' in labour wards, as women wrote in with stories that will be very familiar to those who have studied or experienced birth trauma today.

The tide therefore turned once again with the advent of the 1960s and the theories of 'natural', drug-free childbirth pioneered by Grantly Dick-Read, as described in his book *Childbirth without Fear*. As with chloroform, Dick-Read's innovations were pilloried by the medical establishment. But others, such as the French doctor Fernand Lamaze, took up his ideas and enlarged on them.

Later, in the 1970s, came the modern pain relief techniques we're all familiar with – pethidine, the epidural, and the use of gas and air. But the ideal of a drug-free, completely 'natural' birth didn't go away with these advances. If anything, it became stronger as practitioners such as Janet Balaskas and Sheila Kitzinger advocated 'active birth' in a standing or squatting position, rather than being strapped down on a bed, and doctors became more aware of the importance of bonding between mother and baby immediately after a birth.

These days, it's standard in UK hospitals to put the baby to the mother's breast as soon as he or she is born, if the baby's condition allows it. We can choose a home birth, if our midwives are supportive. In some areas we can choose to go to a midwife-led birth centre. Some hospitals now have these birth centres on site, allowing easy transfer to wards if something goes wrong. We can choose from a multitude of antenatal classes teaching techniques ranging from breathing to hypnotherapy. We have transcutaneous electrical nerve stimulation (TENS) machines, birthing balls, gentle whale music, homoeopathic remedies and birthing pools. Fathers are now welcome in the delivery room. Yet many women still suffer traumatic birth experiences. Our understanding of why this is only just beginning.

How do I know if I have PTSD following childbirth?

The cause may differ but the symptoms of PTSD are similar to those of PTSD following other events. The women I interviewed for this chapter spoke of:

- having flashbacks, nightmares and persistent memories;
- being hospital-phobic;

- feeling determined never to have another baby as they were too afraid;
- being afraid of having sex and of undergoing simple procedures, such as cervical smears or the insertion of a coil;
- feeling intensely guilty – guilty that the birth hadn't been the way they planned, guilty that they had somehow damaged their children by failing to bond with them, guilty that they hadn't somehow lived up to the natural birth ideal.

These are all classic symptoms of PTSD.

A couple of months after I gave birth, I met a friend who had also recently had a child. Her situation was very different from mine. She had gone into labour at 28 weeks. Her child was born weighing just 1 kilogram (2 pounds) and was sent straight to the special care baby unit, where she stayed for the next three months. The baby had to undergo many blood transfusions and medical procedures. There were several instances when my friend did not believe her child would survive.

I couldn't understand why, after all this pain and distress, my friend didn't seem traumatized – whereas I was. Perhaps I was making a fuss about nothing. Perhaps I was being weak. After all, I hadn't sat for days next to my baby wondering if he would live or die. I hadn't given birth so early that my bump was barely showing. I hadn't had to watch my baby go through agonizingly painful medical procedures, or lived with the worry that he would be brain damaged or physically disabled. All that had happened to me was a long, painful birth followed by a hospital stay when my baby had jaundice. What right had I to be traumatized when my friend's problems were so much worse than my own?

I found the answer in the research of Cheryl Beck, Professor of Nursing at the University of Connecticut, USA, who has stated simply: 'Birth trauma is in the eye of the beholder.' Or, put another way, if you found your birth traumatic, then it was a traumatic birth. There is no set amount of blood loss, for example, or agreed level of agony, that 'qualifies' your birth as a traumatic one. As New Zealand midwife and trauma therapist Judy Crompton writes: 'Above all, it needs to be borne in mind that it is the person's perception of the event which traumatizes them, not another person's perceptions of whether an event should or should not be traumatic.'

Nicola

I feel the birth is what caused my postnatal depression. I felt as if I had failed by not being able to give birth properly. I feel it was more like post-traumatic stress.

What causes birth trauma?

It's impossible to say for certain whether or not a woman will experience PTSD after childbirth. However, certain risk factors have emerged, including:

- emergency Caesarean sections and instrumental deliveries;
- fears for the safety of a baby;
- feeling unsupported by one's partner;
- staff who don't keep the woman fully informed of what's happening during or after the birth, or who are dismissive or rude;
- a history of sexual abuse or rape (some experts believe that memories of these experiences can be triggered during the birth of a child);
- pain during the first stages of labour;
- lack of support following the birth;
- stillbirth;
- insufficient aftercare;
- lack of 'control' during labour;
- birth following severe pre-eclampsia;
- birth of a low-birth-weight baby;
- depression during pregnancy;
- ineffective pain relief.

Jane

She [my baby] was whisked off. The only information I got was because my partner went to see her and they told him she was unresponsive and had to be ventilated. I didn't get any more information until 10 o'clock the next morning and I went to see my baby with my partner. The lack of communication between the staff and mums of sick babies was appalling. Nobody offered to take me to see her in the whole time I was immobile. I had to wait for my partner, mum or friend. No calls were made to the ward to find out or let me know of any changes or just her general condition … I still have nightmares. I'm on a bus and I lose my baby. I turn around and she's just not there and I start screaming.

The increased medicalization of birth and what some see as an over-eagerness on the part of surgeons to perform emergency Caesarean deliveries has been cited as one possible cause of the emergence of PTSD. However, it's interesting to note that many women also seem to experience PTSD following a vaginal delivery – one study of 1,550 women found that most of the women who reported trauma symptoms had in fact had a vaginal delivery. It could be that the manner and the environment in which the birth is carried out, rather than the mechanics of the birth, are more important factors in determining whether or not a mother develops PTSD.

Over and over again in my interviews the phrase 'out of control' crops up, both among women who have had a vaginal birth and among those who have had a Caesarean section. To quote the US psychologist Sarah Allen, who interviewed 20 women ten months after giving birth: 'Pain, past experiences and beliefs that their baby would be harmed led to feeling out of control, which was maintained by failed attempts to elicit practical and emotional support from staff and partners.'

Gail
Considering I had major surgery the aftercare was appalling, in an overcrowded and understaffed ward. After leaving theatre I was given no pain relief for almost 24 hours. I had to cry for it and eventually someone noticed. And I am pretty tough.

There have not been, as far as I can ascertain, any studies on the rates of PTSD among mothers who have home births. And because a home birth that is going wrong will transfer to hospital, it would then count as a hospital birth anyway. Certainly the anecdotal evidence suggests that a woman who begins labour at home and is then transferred to hospital is just as much at risk from the factors above as one who has her whole labour in a hospital. However, advocates of home birth say that women who give birth at home are far less likely to experience PTSD and that the main reason why women experience PTSD is because of the risk factors endemic in the hospital environment. These include a higher rate of intervention and the lack of 'control' caused by medical paraphernalia, such as heart-rate monitors that require women to lie still, epidurals that stop women moving around and, of course, the traditional stirrups. It certainly seems true on an anecdotal basis that some women who have suffered PTSD after a first birth have gone on to have successful home births with their second children.

Expectations

What did you expect birth to be like? Chances are it was very different from the reality. A study from Newcastle University found a significant gap between women's expectations of birth and the reality in four areas:

1 the level and type of pain;
2 access to pain relief;
3 the level of participation in and control over decision-making;
4 the level of control during labour.

Some women thought the pain would be an 'all-over' pain; others weren't aware that labour pain comes in 'waves'. Some didn't understand that certain types of pain relief, such as epidurals, would be available only if they gave birth in a hospital rather than in a midwife-led unit or at home. Many didn't realize that the choices that they had made for their birth plan wouldn't necessarily prove practical during labour, and that they wouldn't necessarily be able to make choices during labour.

There's been some debate recently on women who are 'disappointed' with their birth experiences, and who believe their PTSD stems from not getting the birth they wanted. Reactions to this have varied from those who feel that mere 'disappointment' shouldn't be sufficient to trigger PTSD to those who believe that, whatever causes the PTSD, the suffering is just as real.

I fall into the latter camp. I don't believe that women who feel that they have 'failed' or are 'disappointed' by their births are the arrogant 'too-posh-to-push' stereotypes put forward by the media.

For myself, I found that 'failing' to give birth at the birth centre without drugs was a major factor in my PTSD, an experience echoed by several women I interviewed. Perhaps there's a lesson here for those who run antenatal classes and insist that their particular method is 'the best way' to give birth.

Joanne Lally, who carried out the research at Newcastle University discussed above, believes that our disappointment springs from two opposing schools of thought – one that says we shouldn't have to suffer pain in a modern society and one that believes that, because women have been giving birth for thousands of years, we shouldn't necessarily need pain relief. She also says that the popular images of giving birth in five minutes and in full make-up that we see in television dramas and in films, contrasted with the 'horror stories' we hear from friends and parents, conspire to create confusion in our minds about what birth is really like. If you felt like a failure because your labour didn't go to plan, you are not alone and you are not abnormal.

Nicola
Back home, I tried to pretend that everything was all right. I felt terribly lonely and depressed. I had no family nearby to talk to. Whenever I was out, smiling and talking, I felt like I was wearing a mask. I was very tired and disappointed with the way the birth went. I felt I had failed and that I had been failed. After six months, my baby didn't let me breastfeed him any more. I'd failed at that, too.

What are the differences between postnatal depression and PTSD?

Given that both postnatal depression (PND) and PTSD are under-researched areas, it's hardly surprising that we have little understanding of the relationship between the two. However, there does now seem to be a scientific consensus that the two disorders are separate, with the possibility of PND following on from PTSD or PTSD symptoms being a risk factor in the development of PND. The symptoms of PND are discussed in more detail in Chapter 2. However, in brief, they are:

- low mood for prolonged periods of time (a week or more);
- feeling irritable for a lot of the time;

- tearfulness;
- panic attacks;
- difficulty concentrating;
- lack of motivation;
- lack of interest in yourself and your new baby;
- feeling lonely;
- feeling guilty, rejected or inadequate;
- feeling overwhelmed;
- feeling unable to cope;
- difficulty sleeping;
- physical signs of tension, such as headaches, stomach pains or blurred vision.

Recovering from PTSD

In order to recover from PTSD, you must first identify it. It's surprising how many mothers I spoke to had no idea they were suffering from a recognized condition. This isn't surprising. Most of us know about the possibility of PND. It's regularly flagged up in pregnancy books and antenatal classes, and we're therefore more likely to recognize it when it happens to us. It's likely that your partner will also know about PND, and following your birth your health visitor is likely to check that you aren't suffering any PND symptoms. But PTSD is rarely mentioned in pregnancy books or antenatal classes. In fact, you're unlikely to come across it unless you start suspecting and searching.

While screening for PND is commonplace, screening for PTSD is less so. However, Dr Susan Ayers et al. have developed a screening tool for PTSD. The City Birth Trauma Scale is a 29-item questionnaire developed to measure birth-related PTSD according to DSM-5 criteria, which, it is hoped, will lead to better identification of the condition in the future.

Who can I turn to?

If you feel you may have PTSD, start talking. Pick a medical professional you are comfortable with. It may be your doctor, your health visitor or a midwife. Don't let the psychological nature of PTSD put you off talking. You will not be classed as 'mad', and your baby will not be taken away from you. Ask your partner or a trusted friend or relative to come along for moral support if you're scared about going on your own. Write down your symptoms and their frequency so you know exactly what to say. Nerves can have a strange effect on the memory, and your clinician will need to ask you questions.

There are also several dedicated support groups, such as the Birth Trauma Association, which can offer you help and guidance. For details of these groups, see 'Useful contacts' towards the end of this book.

Following a diagnosis of PTSD, you may be offered any of the following options.

Psychotherapy

Psychotherapy is an umbrella term for what most of us know as 'counselling' or 'talking therapies'. Exactly what your psychotherapy involves will depend on what type you're offered. For example, Freudian therapy seeks to make sense of your experience by drawing on your family structure and events that happened in your childhood. Standard counselling involves you talking about your problems to a counsellor, who will work with you to help you find solutions and understand your feelings.

You may also be offered a referral to a cognitive behavioural therapist. Cognitive behavioural therapy (CBT) is a form of psychotherapy that has been found to help some sufferers of PTSD, although as yet there is no published research to support its effectiveness when it is used to deal specifically with women who have PTSD following childbirth. It focuses on how to deal with problems by breaking them down into manageable parts, and it encourages you to examine the way you think and the way you react to certain events.

Several studies have demonstrated that counselling has been useful in helping women overcome bad birth experiences. One study of 348 women found that just a low level of intervention – face-to-face counselling within 72 hours of birth and again via telephone at four to six weeks following birth – resulted in fewer trauma symptoms, a lower risk of depression, a lower risk of stress and lower feelings of self-blame.

When you look for a therapist, ask whether they have experience in dealing with PTSD following childbirth, and make sure they are appropriately qualified.

Debriefing

You may be left with a lot of unanswered questions following your labour. Why did the doctor say what he did? Why was I not offered any pain relief? Why was my baby blue when he or she came out? Why did nobody tell me that my baby wasn't breathing? Why did they need to perform an episiotomy? Having someone to answer these questions and talk you through exactly what happened during the birth can be part of the healing process, and some women find it very helpful in coming to terms with their traumatic labour.

In the UK, you have the right to request your medical records. You can start this process by talking to your GP or health visitor. You can also contact the Patient Liaison Service at the hospital where you gave birth, which should be able to put you in touch with a midwife or doctor who is happy to talk you through exactly what happened during your labour and answer any questions you might have.

It should be noted that the 'debriefing' method is not recommended as a stand-alone therapy under the guidelines produced by the National Institute of Health and Clinical Excellence (NICE). The guidelines state that:

> Single-session formal debriefing focused on the birth should not be routinely offered to women who have experienced a traumatic birth. However, maternity staff and other healthcare professionals should support women who wish to talk about their experience, encourage them to make use of natural support systems available from family and friends, and take into account the effect of the birth on the partner.

So the message seems to be: ensure that you have other forms of support and don't rely on a single briefing to sort you out. It can be useful to talk through your concerns before debriefing with other women who have been through the process on an online support group such as the Birth Trauma Association's Facebook page. Anecdotal evidence suggests that the quality of a debrief is paramount: while some women have found staff to be helpful and supportive, others have found them less so and have felt no better afterwards – and in some cases, they have felt worse.

Antidepressants

You may be offered antidepressants to help you cope with the negative feelings that are a symptom of PTSD. Whether or not you take them is entirely up to you. It is worth bearing in mind that, although they may mask the symptoms, they will not 'cure' your PTSD.

The prospect of taking antidepressants can feel scary and stigmatizing, despite increased awareness of mental health issues in recent years. However, modern antidepressants have helped many thousands of people. Don't dismiss them just because they're 'drugs'. Talk to your GP or health visitor if you have concerns about antidepressants.

You are most likely to be offered one of a class of drugs known as selective serotonin reuptake inhibitors (SSRIs). Like all drugs, these can have side effects. Your doctor will advise you on whether or not it is safe for you to take the drug while breast-feeding. For more information on antidepressants, see Chapter 2.

Eye movement desensitization and reprocessing (EMDR)

This relatively new treatment might sound a little strange, but it has been recognized by the World Health Organization as a treatment for PTSD.

It works by helping you 'process' the traumatic experience. This is achieved by eight phases of treatment, including the Rapid Eye Movement phase, during which you'll be asked to make side-to-side eye movements while recalling the traumatic incident.

It's not exactly understood why EMDR works, but one theory goes that the small eye movements – known as 'visual bilateral stimulation' – help your brain to move on from the traumatic incident that has become 'stuck' in your brain.

There is not a great deal of evidence around using EMDR specifically for PTSD following childbirth, and more research needs to be done on just how effective it is. However, anecdotally, it does seem to have helped some women.

In conclusion

From my own experience – again reflected in that of the women I interviewed for this chapter – I found that well-meaning friends, relatives and medical professionals initially fell back on one of three well-worn clichés when I tried to talk about my birth trauma:

- 'You'll forget the pain.'
- 'You've got a healthy baby – what are you worried about?'
- 'You should have had a home birth' / 'You should have gone to a birth centre' / 'You should have chosen/refused an epidural.'

'You'll forget the pain.'

This may indeed be true of the vast majority of women – after all, why else would we go on to have more children? And if you've ever experienced a serious injury, you may well look back and have no memory of exactly how you felt when you broke your leg. Unfortunately, and as research has shown, women who have PTSD do not forget the pain. They replay it endlessly, they dream about it and some find it so overwhelming that they refuse to have any more children.

Few would imply to someone who had undergone a major traumatic event such as a car accident that they will 'forget the pain'. I suggest that the same consideration should be extended towards women suffering from PTSD following childbirth. It is important to realize that there is nothing 'wrong' with you if you don't conform to the accepted norm. So your mother-in-law had six children, was in agony for all of them but forgot all about it. That's great news for her, but it has nothing to do with your experience.

'You've got a healthy baby – what are you worried about?'

I was lucky. I had a healthy baby. Some of the women I interviewed were not so lucky, and we have already seen that having a stillbirth or a low-birth-weight baby are risk factors for PTSD. But it would seem from the research that other risk factors such as levels of support and the birth environment are equally important. Just because your baby is healthy does not mean that you can't be suffering from PTSD. PTSD is something that you suffer, not your baby. It's worth saying it once again: birth trauma is in the eye of the beholder.

'You should have had a home birth' / 'You should have gone to a birth centre' / 'You should have chosen/refused an epidural.'

Dwelling on what you should or should not have done is unlikely to make you feel better. Many women with PTSD cite a lack of control and a lack of choice as part of their birth experiences. It is difficult, for example, to 'choose' an epidural when you are experiencing pain worse than you have ever felt before. It is difficult to 'choose' a home birth or a birth centre if, like me, you went into labour early or your baby is likely to be breech. Sometimes, circumstances make it impossible to have the birth you wanted. Accepting that and moving on are part of the recovery process. You are unlikely to be helped by people who want to claim your PTSD as proof or otherwise of their own convictions about birth.

The important thing to remember is that PTSD is not your fault. It is a natural reaction to a traumatic event. It is not something that can be dismissed just because you happen to be lucky in another respect. There's nothing wrong with counting your blessings, and it could be that by comparing yourself to other women who are not lucky enough to have healthy babies you will end up feeling better. However, this is more likely to make you dwell on your own perceived inadequacies. ('She had a much worse time than me and her baby has heart problems, yet she's coping fine … I must be weak – or cowardly or ungrateful – to feel like this.')

You are not weak, cowardly or ungrateful. You are a normal person experiencing an understandable reaction to a traumatic event involving both yourself and your baby. Many women have gone on to give birth again and have better experiences. You are not alone and you can recover.

Eleanor
Talk to someone, anyone, before it eats you up and ruins what should be a very happy time or recurs in later life.

2
Postnatal depression and puerperal psychosis

During my pregnancy, I remember saying airily to my husband, 'Oh yes, and the symptoms of PND are this and this and this, but don't worry, I'm not really the sort of person to get PND.' To me, PND was something that happened to other women – women with abusive partners, perhaps. Or single mothers having to cope on their own. Or women without supportive families. Or women who hadn't planned their pregnancies. Certainly, I thought, PND couldn't happen to someone like me.

I was, of course, spectacularly wrong about this (and about plenty of other things). The truth is, of course, that PND can happen to anyone. It can happen to your next-door neighbour, it can happen to Brooke Shields. It can happen to a jobless single mother living in a council flat and to a multimillionaire City executive with an eight-bedroom house in Hampstead. PND is an illness, and, like any other illness, it does not discriminate.

A friend of mine who suffered with severe depression linked to myalgic encephalopathy (ME) once remarked to me that the funny thing about the depression hole is that everything makes perfect sense while you're in it. She was right. To me, it made perfect sense that my friends no longer liked me, that I was a terrible mother and an awful person, that everyone would be much better off if I wasn't there any more. There was no perspective in my hole, which is why it was so hard to get help. Why did I need help? I was clearly suffering because I was a terrible person, and no doctor could help me with that, surely?

After six months of this, my husband insisted that I see my GP, who diagnosed PND and offered me antidepressants. I declined, more out of fear than logic, and ended up attending group therapy run on Freudian lines. We all sat around discussing our childhoods and our parents and our lives, while our babies played happily in the middle of our circle. I'm still not entirely sure whether or not it cured my PND. But it was good to know that I wasn't alone.

It's hardly surprising that we are fearful about admitting to PND. A storyline on *Coronation Street*, one of the UK's most-watched soap operas, featured a woman suffering from PND returning her baby to the hospital in which he was born and claiming that he couldn't be her child. She then pushed her baby's pram in front of a moving car and was sectioned under the Mental Health Act.

It is safe to say that this does not reflect the average woman's experience of PND, and it's not ridiculous to suppose that portrayals of this nature play a large part in why so many women don't report PND. Indeed, many of us make a conscious decision to hide it, determined to put a brave face on it, determined to show how brilliantly we are coping.

I had a few idle moments recently and decided to clear out my email Sent box. I hadn't looked at it since before my son was born. I didn't get very far: fascinated, I reread the emails I'd sent at those times when I'd been seriously considering suicide. You'd never know. They're full of jaunty phrases – 'Getting used to sleepless nights!! Oh well!' and endless references to how gorgeous and lovely and clever my baby is.

Reading these emails, I wondered why I'd gone to such incredible lengths to cover up what I was feeling. I suppose, like most people, I'd been ashamed of my PND. And I'd felt that it was my duty to get over it by myself, that I should be able to 'cope' – whatever that means. If 'coping' means 'not actually killing myself', well, yes, I 'coped'. But I wished I had sought help sooner. This chapter aims to help you understand exactly what PND is, how it can be treated, and how you can get help.

Alison

I wasn't really aware I had PND until quite recently, after speaking to friends and having time to reflect on the past few years. After having my daughter, I completed an Edinburgh Postnatal Depression Scale questionnaire, which is used to help diagnose PND, as part of research being done by the medical centre I was attending. It showed indications of PND, and I was asked if I wanted anyone to talk to. At the time, I put the daily tears down to tiredness and having two children quite close together, so I said I was fine.

As well as crying at least once or twice a day, I felt I was letting my older child down if I didn't go out and attend groups or meet people, but the hassle of getting both young ones out also reduced me to tears. I felt very resentful towards my daughter for changing the 'perfect' time I'd had with her brother before she was born and these feelings of resentment then led to feelings of guilt. None of this was helped by her waking up between four and five times a night until she was two, and my husband being unable to provide any practical help in the week due to his job. Weekends were spent with one of us trying to catch up on sleep while the other looked after the children, so I never really talked to him about it.

When she was two, my daughter started sleeping through the night. It took a couple of months, but I started to notice how much easier things were becoming. I stopped crying at every little thing that upset or frustrated me, and I started to see my daughter as a lovable little girl rather than an annoyance. I have just given up my part-time job to look after her full time because I feel I missed out on her first two years of life. I have all these memories of my son at different ages, what he was wearing or doing or saying; I have none of those of my daughter.

I wish I had taken up the offer of help when it was made instead of thinking PND was for women who couldn't cope with motherhood. I wanted to be a 'super-mum' who could juggle children and a job and still be blissfully happy!

What is PND?

PND is generally defined as non-psychotic depression that occurs during a specific time period after a baby is born. Although the definition of the 'official' time period during which depression can be said to be 'postnatal' varies, it is generally accepted that PND can appear up to three months following chidlbirth, but some studies have found it occurring more than six months after the birth, although the World Health Organization's time period is six weeks. Health professionals need to bear these recommended periods in mind when making a diagnosis. As NICE points out in its guidelines for professionals, PND can be used as 'a label for any mental illness occurring postnatally', meaning that other serious conditions might be missed by a doctor too quick to assume PND.

It's estimated that 10–15 per cent of new mothers suffer some kind of depressive illness. However, as with all mental illnesses, the actual prevalence could be much higher. A 2011 survey of 2,318 mothers undertaken by the charity 4Children estimated that around three in ten new mothers may experience PND. It also found that approximately 25 per cent of mothers were still suffering PND up to a year after their child was born – and that more than half (58 per cent) did not seek help.

What are the symptoms?

One question I've often encountered from mothers who haven't suffered from PND is how on earth you tell the difference between PND and the 'normal' feelings and challenges encountered by new mothers. After all, who isn't exhausted, depressed and unable to concentrate when they have a month-old baby in the house? There's no easy answer: just like depression that isn't linked to birth, symptoms vary hugely, and every woman is different. However, PND is distinct from what's known as the 'baby blues' – feeling low, tearful and exhausted in the first week following childbirth – which is experienced by around 80 per cent of mothers. As a basic guide, standard depression symptoms may include:

- low mood for prolonged periods of time (a week or more);
- feeling irritable for a lot of the time;
- tearfulness;
- panic attacks or feeling worried, upset or agitated for no particular reason;
- difficulty concentrating;
- lack of motivation – losing interest in your normal daily life and things you enjoyed previously;
- feeling lonely;
- feeling guilty, rejected or inadequate;
- feeling overwhelmed and having difficulty making decisions, even ones that previously seemed very simple;
- losing your appetite;
- having difficulty concentrating;

- feeling unable to cope;
- difficulty sleeping even when you're exhausted;
- physical signs of tension, such as headaches, stomach pains or blurred vision;
- having thoughts about suicide or death.

Symptoms specific to PND generally involve your baby in some way. For example, you might feel that you can't look after your baby properly. You might think about harming yourself or the baby. You might feel angry at yourself for feeling this way or convinced that having a baby was a huge mistake. Many mothers have described feeling 'trapped' or 'out of control'. You might have obsessive thoughts or compulsive behaviour such as washing your hands over and over again. You might suffer from extreme anxiety, convinced that your baby is going to die or become ill. Or your baby might make you anxious, to the extent that you can't even bear to be in the same room as him or her. You might have a terrible sense of loss, that you've missed out on what everyone tells you is supposed to be a wonderful time with your baby. Or you could feel that you've lost your 'self', your personality and your old life.

An interesting and possibly under-reported aspect of PND that came from the women I spoke to was one of feeling incredibly overprotective of their babies, to the extent that they were too scared to let others even hold or touch them. One woman told mc that this fceling had convinced her that she didn't have PND, since she thought that only mothers who didn't want to be with their babies could have the condition.

Another common symptom is feeling very alone. You may think that you're the only woman to have this condition. You may worry that, if you seek help, you'll be labelled 'mad' and have your children taken away – indeed, I have seen many women citing this very myth on parenting websites. If you feel like this, please remember that you are not alone. There are thousands of women just like you, and nobody is going to take your baby away because you have PND. It is true that some women need to be admitted to hospital with PND, but these cases are very rare.

Amanda

I think my PND first showed itself when my daughter was four months old. She used to sleep in my bed, and I would turn and look at her and ask her if I could keep her. I honestly didn't think at the time I could have PND, as I was overly protective towards her. I wouldn't let anyone else look after her and was cautious about who I let into the house. I would get tearful and panicky as I thought someone was going to take her away from me. I didn't really talk to anyone about how I was feeling as I thought it was normal and it would go away in time – I just had to convince myself that nobody was going to take her away. I was more concerned that my parents thought I had a problem. I didn't see the problem myself.

Paula

I had the baby blues but they didn't seem to go away. I had terrible memory loss, even forgetting the date and time my daughter was born. I cried all the time. I couldn't make my daughter's bottles up – I thought I would infect her and I could never remember how many spoonfuls I put into the bottles so I had to tip them out and start again. I didn't want to go out anywhere unless my mum was with me. I had panic attacks and had dreams that my baby would get stolen or I would poison her or drop her by accident. I wanted to run away or jump out the window, but I decided that wherever I went my daughter would come with me. It was me and her together. I was very protective of her.

I was married at the time but didn't feel I had the support of my husband. I spoke to my mum. I practically lived with Mum as I didn't want to be on my own. She picked me up nearly every day. My mother-in-law told me it was a phase and couldn't understand what I was going through. My friend told me to snap out of it. After having a baby of her own she understands more. I felt that I only had my mum and my sister at the time. After a few months I did get to know my neighbour who had recently had a baby and she had PND too, so we used to get together and share our problems. That was fantastic and the support I needed but unfortunately she moved away.

How is PND diagnosed?

Your health visitor, GP or midwife should be on the lookout for possible PND symptoms from the moment you give birth. However, as in any aspect of healthcare, not every practitioner is geared up to recognize PND symptoms, though in general medical professionals are far more aware and sympathetic than they used to be. Unfortunately the number of health visitors, traditionally the people quickest to spot PND, is falling. Evidence submitted to a parliamentary inquiry in October 2018 by the Institute of Health Visiting (IHV) found that numbers dropped by 20 per cent between October 2015 and April 2018. If you think you have PND, you need to see a medical professional as soon as possible. PND can go away on its own, but, equally, it can be cured and there is no need to suffer in silence.

There is a significant difference between PND and what's known (rather cloyingly, in my opinion) as the 'baby blues'. (This deceptively cute-sounding name doesn't, in my experience, come anywhere close to describing the mood swings that arrive after giving birth.) In general, the 'baby blues' – feeling weepy, unsettled, depressed and miserable after the baby is born – will go away after a couple of weeks. PND will not. According to NICE guidelines, you should be assessed for PND if you have symptoms of the 'baby blues' that haven't improved after ten to 14 days.

NICE says that you should also be asked the following questions when you first see someone about your pregnancy, when you first see a midwife, and again usually four to six weeks and three to four months after you have given birth. These questions will help pick up signs of depression.

- During the past month, have you often been bothered by feeling down, depressed or hopeless?
- During the past month, have you often been bothered by having little interest or pleasure in doing things?

Depending on your answers, you may also be asked:

- Is this something you feel you need or want help with?

If your answers suggest that you may have depression, you may be asked to fill in a questionnaire. This is usually the Edinburgh Postnatal Depression Scale, which is used to help diagnose PND. It's a questionnaire that you fill out around six to eight weeks after the birth of your baby, and it is designed to pick up symptoms of PND. You'll be asked to fill it in on the basis of how you have felt over the last seven days. Your 'score' will show whether or not you are showing symptoms of PND.

What causes PND?

Nobody really knows what causes PND. But it would appear it is a condition that can be found worldwide. A recent review of the available literature found PND to be prevalent in more than 40 countries, from Taiwan to Brazil. In some countries, such as Austria, the prevalence was very low. In others, such as Chile and South Africa, the prevalence was much higher.

A number of factors make it more likely that you'll get PND. They include:

- having had PND before – one study puts the risk of recurrence at 25 per cent;
- lack of social support – for example, being a single mother, having an unsupportive or abusive partner or not having any family or friends in your area;
- having a baby who is premature or ill in some way;
- your mother's dying when you were a child;
- having had other recent stressful life events such as bereavement, moving house or losing your job;
- having had another depressive illness in the past or having been depressed during your pregnancy.

Will my having PND affect my baby in later life?

The honest answer to this question is: once again, we simply don't know. Several studies seem to show that PND can adversely affect children's mood, although researchers are at pains to point out the flaws in these pieces of research: namely, that it's very difficult to 'measure' both adult and child moods accurately. A small study of 149 women found that the children of women who were depressed three months after giving birth had lower IQ scores, and one of 40 depressed women and 48 non-depressed women found that male children seemed to be more vulnerable to the effects of their mothers' moods. But a study of 1,329 German women who suffered from depression and their children found 'negligible' effects on the cognitive development of the children.

This is just a small selection of the studies that have attempted to answer this question. Knowledge is power but in this case, until medical science has a definitive answer – which, let's face it, may not happen for a while, if ever – it's best to try not to worry about how your PND might be affecting your child. As with so many aspects of depressive illness, there is little conclusive evidence one way or the other and so much depends on individual circumstances and the personality of the mother and child. The best thing you can do for yourself and your child is to seek help as soon as possible.

Treatments for PND

In an ideal world, every woman experiencing PND would be offered a choice of treatments, including counselling and drug treatment if needed. However, we know that women with PND do not always get the treatment they need.

Well-meaning family and friends may think they're helping by telling you to 'snap out of it' or that PND is 'normal' and that 'it'll wear off in time'. Of course, people with any kind of depression cannot choose to suddenly feel better. Depression is an illness, and, like any other illness, it needs treatment.

There are two main forms of treatment for PND: counselling and drug therapy. All women are different, and what works for one might not work for another. Whatever treatment you choose, it's important to find out as much as you can about it. Don't be afraid to ask your GP – that's what he or she is there for, and when it comes to something as important as treatment for PND, there's no such thing as a 'stupid question'.

Louise
Having had depression before, I knew the signs. So I spoke with my husband and my mother, then went straight to the doctor. My concern was that I needed to be well for my baby, but I also needed 'me' back too.

Drug treatment

Your GP may offer you one of several antidepressants if you are diagnosed with PND. The most common antidepressants in use today belong to a class of drugs known as selective serotonin reuptake inhibitors (SSRIs). These drugs work by increasing the levels of the neurotransmitter serotonin in your brain. This chemical is one thought to affect the way your brain works. These are not addictive, and it may take several weeks before they start working.

Your doctor should ask you if you are breastfeeding, since some drugs pass into your breast milk. Fluoxetine, for example, isn't recommended for breastfeeding mothers, but sertraline and paroxetine should be fine, because they pass into the milk in only extremely small amounts.

There's not a great deal of research on antidepressants and their effect on PND. Studies have tended to be small and to have a high drop-out rate. However, SSRIs are also used for different kinds of depression, not just PND, and they have been found to be effective.

There is certainly a stigma attached to taking antidepressants. But it's important to remember that PND is an illness. You wouldn't think twice about taking antibiotics for an infection or an aspirin for a headache. Try to look at drug therapy in the same way. One study investigated how women with PND felt about their drug treatment. Several made comments such as 'I'm not a tablet taker' or 'I don't like taking tablets ... they are bound to do you more harm in the long run.' I found that women that I talked to for this chapter also used similar phrases. It's perfectly understandable to have these fears. Remember, nobody is forcing you to take tablets. But it is vital to keep your doctor informed of any decisions you make about your medication, because coming off antidepressants suddenly could be dangerous.

The SSRIs that you might be prescribed are discussed below.

Fluoxetine (brand name: Prozac)

In one study of fluoxetine for PND, researchers found 'highly significant improvements' in depressed women who were given the drug plus cognitive behavioural therapy counselling sessions.

The women who took fluoxetine improved more than the women given a placebo. Frequently reported side effects of fluoxetine include headaches, nervousness, nausea and diarrhoea. Drowsiness, rash and sexual dysfunction can occur, although these side effects are rare.

Paroxetine (brand name: Seroxat)

A study of 35 depressed women who took paroxetine also found a significant improvement in symptoms. The women were split into two groups, one group receiving just paroxetine and the other group also receiving counselling sessions. The researchers found no major statistical differences between the two groups. Frequently reported side effects include nausea, sweating, drowsiness and dizziness. Rarer side effects include nervousness, anxiety, agitation, rash, itching, hives, joint pain, weight loss and convulsions.

Sertraline (brand name: Lustral)

There have been very few studies specifically on sertraline for PND. However, a small study of 14 women found that those who took sertraline seemed less likely to suffer a recurrence of PND than those who took a placebo. Frequently reported side effects include nausea, diarrhoea, loss of appetite, indigestion and sleep problems. Rarer side effects include dizziness, tremor, confusion, palpitations, fainting and rash.

Other SSRIs

You might also be offered fluvoxamine (brand name: Faverin) or citalopram (brand name: Cipramil). These have been studied widely in the context of general depression in adults but haven't been investigated significantly for women suffering from PND.

Paula

I went to the doctor and told him my symptoms, and he put me on tablets straight away, although I was reluctant to take them. I tried several different medications before they found the right one for me. I think I ended up taking citalopram. They did help. You feel worse when you start taking them, but then they do help. Although I never really felt myself on them. I didn't really have any emotions on them. I couldn't cry or laugh. Maybe that was just me at the time, I don't know.

Leila

My husband told me one day over the phone that he thought I was depressed, and on the same day a girl at work told me to go to see a doctor, so I did. She told me to wait for a week to think things through and if I felt that I wanted something she would give me something. I took Prozac for a month and a bit, but then felt that I wanted to try to go it alone. It helped immensely. I didn't like the idea of taking anything, as I feel I am a person in control of things and to feel that I lost control was not good for me. But the tablets helped tons, and I felt good, and they allowed me to tackle normal situations. I have been off them now for a while and sometimes I get moody again but have learned to curb how I feel because I know now what it is.

A note on hormone treatment

There is very little research on whether hormone treatment can make a difference to PND. One small study of 61 depressed women treated with the hormone oestrogen found that the hormone seemed to work better than a placebo. But this study isn't enough to suggest that PND can be cured with hormone treatment.

What about alternative therapies?

There's very little research on the effectiveness of therapies such as yoga, light therapy, aromatherapy and massage. However, they're unlikely to do you any harm, and if they help to relax you and give you a break from your childcare responsibilities, then there's no reason why you shouldn't use them. Do bear in mind, though, that herbal remedies, although 'natural', can also be extremely strong and could interact with drugs you are taking for other conditions. Make sure you check with your doctor before taking any herbal medicines.

You might have heard of St John's wort, a herb that has been found to be effective in treating depression in adults. There hasn't been any research on whether or not St John's wort helps PND, and you shouldn't take it while you're pregnant or breastfeeding. If you're planning to take it, make sure you let your doctor know.

Talking therapies

As many women with PND don't want to take drugs, it makes sense to consider other kinds of therapy. Broadly speaking, there are two main kinds of talking therapy that have been used to treat PND: psychotherapy and cognitive behavioural therapy.

There are no clear lines of distinction between these two therapies, and many different schools of thought within them, so the following is very much a rough guide. In general, both will involve talking about your thoughts and emotions.

Both of these types of talking therapy have been found to be effective in studies, although, as ever with PND, there isn't a great deal of research available. In general, individual therapy sessions seem be more effective than group therapy. But this can all depend on what kind of person you are.

Psychotherapy or counselling

A psychotherapist or counsellor will work with you to help you to understand your relationships – within and outside your family – and your conflicts. You may have to talk about things that upset you or things that you found traumatic. You may have to think about things from the past that you've tried to forget about, but you'll also be encouraged to find ways of dealing with your feelings.

Cognitive behavioural therapy

Cognitive behavioural therapy is all about helping you to change the way you behave. The method tries to break your old habits of thinking and 'rewire' your brain into reacting differently to events. Your counsellor will work with you to identify these negative patterns. Once you're able to do that, you can start working on how to break them.

Advantages and disadvantages of talking therapies

The world can be a very lonely place when you become a mother for the first time. Sometimes it helps just having a designated time with someone to talk about your thoughts and feelings. These therapies also don't have the side effects associated with drugs, and they won't affect your ability to breastfeed.

However, therapy is not for everyone. You may feel very uncomfortable talking about your feelings and reliving your experiences. You may not get on with your therapist. You may not be able to access paid-for treatment. Or you may find that the demands of your baby, job and home don't fit in with the therapist's schedule.

You are likely to be in a highly vulnerable state and you need someone you can trust, so only ever use therapists who are registered with a recognized national body. (See 'Useful contacts' for more details on finding a therapist.)

Amanda

I eventually asked for help when I realized I hadn't been outside my front door in almost two months. I asked my mum and she came round with the health visitor. I was offered tablets at first and was put on Cipramil as I was still feeding my daughter myself. I honestly think it didn't help. I felt happier and would go out more, but I still wouldn't let anyone look after my daughter and would get panicky if my parents had her for any length of time. I eventually went back to my doctor and explained how I was feeling and was asked if counselling would help me get to the bottom of my PND. I found out a lot about myself through this, and it really helped more than the drugs did as I now understand the cause of my PND.

Paula

My doctor suggested that I go to a local baby massage class to get to know other mums, but I hated it. I felt that they were all looking at me and judging me. It would have been better to go to a class or a meeting for other mums with PND, but unfortunately at the time there was nothing around.

Some other ways you can help yourself

The following suggestions are purely anecdotal. They may not help you but they certainly won't do you any harm.

Create a support network for yourself and your baby. Find mother and baby groups, identify potentially helpful relatives or join classes. Having PND makes all these normal things a lot harder. I remember being too terrified to go to any groups because I was afraid the other mothers would all be perfect. If you feel like this, try a class such as baby massage or baby swimming. You won't be under any pressure to talk and you can get to know people slowly.

Attempt to get out of the house at least once a day. Yes, it seems to take for ever just to gather up all your baby's nappies, bottles and so on, and when the weather's horrible it's so much easier to sit and stare at the walls. But getting out, even if it's just a short walk to the park, will clear your head and remind you that there is a world out there.

Talk to people about how you feel. We are not superwomen, although we would like to be. Sometimes, however much we would like to cope, we simply can't. There's no shame in that. Again and again, I've spoken to women who felt too ashamed to admit they were feeling depressed and wished they had sought help earlier.

Don't be afraid to ask for, and accept, help. Many women I've spoken to felt worried about asking for help because they thought their condition wasn't serious enough – that they had healthy babies, so they should be grateful and keep quiet. There is no need to compare yourself to anyone else. Think about yourself and how you are feeling.

Partners and PND

Having a partner with PND can be a terrifying experience. It is hard to watch the woman you love and who bore your child turn into a stranger during a period that is supposed to be the happiest of your lives. Now, more than ever, she needs the support, patience and love of her partner.

You, the partner, may feel helpless, but in fact you may well be the biggest help of all. Often it is partners who notice that something is wrong and encourage the mother to take that vital first step to go to her doctor. If you suspect that your partner has PND, try to talk to her during a time when she's not likely to be stressed or upset (for example, bath time, feeding time and a nappy change are all times to be avoided). Wait until the baby is sleeping, then talk to her. Don't steam in – be gentle. Suggest that you both go to the doctor. It might help to print out some information on PND from the internet or to show her this book. Reassure her that you love her and that you want to help and support her in the treatment choices she makes.

The future

It may seem impossible at the moment, but there is life after PND. With the right treatment and the right support, you can recover. This condition does not have to blight the rest of your life. You are not a freak, you are not a bad person and you can put this behind you.

It's true that having PND once means you're more at risk of having it a second time. However, it's also true that many women who have had PND in a first pregnancy go on to have more children and don't suffer again. It's also worth bearing in mind that, if you do decide to have another child, your GP, midwife and health visitor will all be alert to the fact that you have had PND and will be able to pick up on the early signs.

Sarah
Do go and seek help, even though you may feel like you are wasting the doctor's time. You are not, and you are not the only mum that feels bad. Take gentle exercise (I did yoga and Pilates, and they are still my 'sanity break') and love yourself – you are not a bad mother no matter how negative you feel. I also made myself go out and do things with my daughter to get me out of the house. I worked on the basis that I'd paid to do a course of some sort with her so I was going to go, as money was precious, so I felt very determined about it. Don't be afraid of taking medication. If it doesn't help straight away, then maybe a different type might be needed. Essentially, be brave and try to communicate how you feel. This was vital for me and if I'd had a bad day I'd say so to my husband so we could give each other space and support.

Amanda
My only advice is to seek help. If you're not happy going alone, then take a friend or family member. And don't ever think there must be 'something wrong with you'. There isn't – you've just got a horrible illness that robs you of the most special time in your life.

What is puerperal psychosis?

Puerperal psychosis is a rare but extremely serious disorder also known as postnatal or postpartum psychosis. It's not the same as PND and requires very different treatment. It affects around one in 1,000 mothers. It's believed to be a reaction to the changes in hormone levels resulting from childbirth, although it has also been linked to genetic factors. It's not yet known why some women get it and some don't, and there's not a great deal of research on the subject. However, if you've had a mental illness before you got pregnant, you're at higher risk of getting puerperal psychosis.

Puerperal psychosis usually starts soon after you have given birth. Symptoms may include:

- hallucinations;
- delusions, which may involve harming the baby or yourself;
- violent mood swings, going from elated to depressed in a matter of minutes;
- extremely irrational behaviour, such as reckless spending, binge-eating or dangerous driving.

If you have not had puerperal psychosis before, you will not necessarily be aware that anything is wrong. In many cases, it is partners, family members or medical professionals who pick up that a new mother is behaving strangely, although some women are able to recognize that what they're feeling is not right. If you or your partner have any suspicions that you might be suffering from puerperal psychosis or recognize the symptoms listed above, it is essential that professional medical help is sought as quickly as possible, because both mother and baby are at risk of harm.

If you have had it before, make sure that your partner, GP, midwife and health visitor know about it. They should be keeping a very close eye on you. Educate your partner and family about the symptoms so they can be on the alert if it happens again.

With the right treatment, puerperal psychosis can be cured. Generally, it will be treated with a combination of anti-psychotic drugs and antidepressants. Mothers and babies are usually admitted to hospital for treatment. Electroconvulsive therapy may also be used if symptoms are particularly severe.

Puerperal psychosis is a terrifying illness that can have huge repercussions for the whole family. In one study, mothers who suffered spoke of their feelings of loss, guilt and grief. They felt that those first precious weeks with their child had been sullied. Some were afraid that they had somehow affected their child adversely. Recovery from puerperal psychosis can be a slow process and you should not be afraid to seek counselling and support if you feel you need it.

3
Learning to love your baby

Bonding is supposed to be the great birth guarantee. No matter how difficult your pregnancy, no matter how protracted your labour, you can look forward to a lovely cuddly bonding session with your baby at the end of it. At least, that was the impression I got. During my pregnancy, I asked a lot of people what it had been like seeing their babies for the first time. They all agreed: wonderful, amazing, fantastic. They talked of a 'great wave' of love on seeing their son or daughter for the first time; a 'rush' of adoration, something mystical and beautiful. Naturally, this was something I looked forward to. So I was pretty shocked when, for me, it simply didn't happen.

Perhaps it was the 20-hour labour, perhaps it was the various drugs swirling around my brain, perhaps it was something deeper going on in my unconscious mind. Perhaps it was that I'd been told the pain would stop as soon as I gave birth (it didn't). But it will remain one of the biggest regrets of my life that my first words to my son were, 'Get him off me, please.' So my little boy spent his first five minutes on this earth being held by his dad while the midwives stitched me up.

I felt nothing for my son for a long time. But it was my job as a mother to look after him, and I'd always prided myself on doing a job well. So I kept him clean and fed and spent all day with a fixed grin on my face in case he saw me looking sad and realized the truth. But I seemed to have no maternal instinct. Friends talked of 'knowing' their babies. I didn't know mine: there was no knowing him. Everything he did seemed completely random. He was white noise: I couldn't tune in to him.

An example: my husband and I took him for a routine blood test when he was a few weeks old, in order to check that the jaundice he'd suffered as a newborn was subsiding. In the waiting room, he started to cry. I remember saying to my husband, 'He's crying, what shall we do?' My husband simply picked his son out of the buggy and cuddled him. He stopped crying. That hadn't even occurred to me. What kind of mother was I, a mother that couldn't even work out that her baby needed a cuddle?

I know that I love my son more than anything – now. But I'm still not sure exactly when I started to love him. I've read that other mothers with bonding problems have had this blinding flash of realization, a moment when they've fallen madly in love with their baby. But it wasn't like that for me. I sometimes think of that love like a lost file on my computer: perhaps it was always there, it just took a while to find out where it was, what it was called, and how to access it.

What is bonding?

Bonding is fascinating, it is hugely complicated and it is as yet insufficiently explained by science. There has been a huge amount of research on bonding in both animals and humans, and a great deal of speculation as to exactly what bonding is, how it happens and why, sometimes, it doesn't happen.

The dictionary definition of bonding is 'the process by which individuals become emotionally attached to one another'. That's so wide as to be more or less meaningless. But it gives us a good starting point and mentions an important issue – bonding, although it is often presented as an instant development, is actually a process that's begun way before the birth. It's something that evolves, not something that just appears.

In fact, it's likely that bonding starts as soon as you know you're pregnant. If you've given up smoking, drinking, eating unpasteurized cheese and bungee jumping while you're pregnant, you're making sacrifices for the health of your unborn child. Therefore, you're emotionally attached to it. You're likely to get more attached as the unborn child becomes more 'real' – anecdotally, I've often heard stories of mothers (and especially fathers) only really coming to terms with the fact that a baby is on the way when they see the first image of their baby at the three-month scan. Later, feeling the baby move and kick, seemingly in response to your voice or other stimulation, helps your image of your child to become stronger. One study of 481 pregnant women found that, by the seventh month of pregnancy, two-thirds of the women had developed a strong maternal bond.

Bonding could be a chemical process, too. A recent study measured levels of the hormone oxytocin in pregnant women. When the women gave birth, the researchers measured their levels of bonding. The results showed that the women with higher levels of oxytocin during early pregnancy carried out far more bonding activities, such as looking at, touching and playing with their baby, than the women with lower levels of the hormone.

Bonding is a lot more than just feeling love – it's showing it as well. Once your baby is born, you carry out bonding actions unconsciously. Talking to your baby, playing with your baby, touching and kissing your baby all help to let your baby know that you are his or her mother. He or she will respond to you with little noises and movements, even though you might not be aware of them. A bond is a two-way process. So even if you might not feel full of love, you can still let your baby know that you're there.

What happens when you don't bond?

Around 29 per cent of women diagnosed with PND have bonding issues. There are many shades on the bonding spectrum. If you don't bond with your baby, you may feel indifferent to him or her. You may experience feelings of hatred, extreme irritation or indifference. You might find it impossible to look after or to interact with your baby. You might feel afraid – almost baby-phobic. In extreme cases, you might also want to harm your baby. If this is the case, you need to get help as soon as possible. (See the section 'Hurting or neglecting your baby' at the end of this chapter.) These feelings can start as soon as the baby has been born, or later. They are likely to be compounded by feelings of guilt that you're not responding to your baby the way society expects you to.

Amy
At five weeks, I lost it. She had just been sick on me following a late-night feed, and I had to call my husband to come and sort her out. I handed her over and walked away, got myself cleaned up and then got into the spare bed. I spent all night sobbing, and in the morning I had to beg my husband not to go to work as I didn't want to be alone with her. I couldn't bring myself to look at her, let alone pick her up. I left my husband to do everything for her. I didn't want to hurt her at all – that never even entered my head – but I knew I didn't want her. I even asked my husband to call social services to come and take her away. He refused, of course!

A special maternal bond?

We are generally brought up with the idea that the maternal bond is special: there is no bond like it, and if something happens to break that bond, then the child will suffer. This could have its root in the work of Dr John Bowlby in the early 1950s. Bowlby's theory of maternal deprivation held that the relationship of a mother and child was unique and that the child would suffer serious consequences if the bond was broken. He believed that this bonding had to take place within the first six months of a child's life.

The theory came in for serious criticism but has also been used many times since to 'prove' political and social theories, especially regarding women in the workplace. Bowlby later amended his theory, and it's now generally accepted that a child can be cared for by the mother or father – or, indeed, a grandparent or an adoptive parent – with no ill effects. There is certainly no evidence that fathers are any less good at caring for their children than mothers.

However, the original Bowlby theory still lingers on in the collective unconscious, reinforced by the thousands of images, words and examples of women as 'natural' carers and nurturers that we see from birth. Every time you worry that you're somehow 'unnatural', every time you're convinced that you should have bonded with your baby instantly and that your failure to do so has damaged your child, chances are that it's Bowlby's theory echoing down the generations. There is no need to feel guilty if you didn't instantly bond with your child or you've experienced bonding problems. It's perfectly normal, it doesn't mean you're a terrible mother or a bad person, and it's unlikely to have a permanent effect on your baby.

Amy
All I could think of was that this thing had come into our lives and had taken over. I knew having a baby wouldn't be easy, but I never expected just how terrible it would feel. What also didn't help was, because she was an IVF baby, everyone kept telling me that I must love her so much more because of what we went through. The trouble was I didn't! I just wanted my life back where I knew what I was doing. I wanted to go back to my job, which I loved. I certainly didn't want to be a mother any more!

Jo
I felt numb. I didn't really understand why I felt that way. Because my daughter was planned I felt like I had to bond with her straight away. I also felt very guilty for feeling that way. I hated myself for being a bad mother and even now I still feel the guilt.

Why didn't I bond with my baby?

Nobody knows why some women develop a bond instantly and some don't. We can identify a few risk factors, however. It makes sense that you might have more problems bonding if your baby is born early or is unwell. A study by Stern discusses the conflict between the psychological pregnancy and the physical one, the moment when the 'imagined' baby becomes the 'real' baby. Few pregnant women don't idly speculate about what their baby will be like, and not many of us imagine our 'dream' baby with a heart condition or a cleft palate. But few of us get any warning that we are likely to have a premature or sick baby. Although scans can indicate some conditions, such as Down's syndrome, they are not always accurate and there are many conditions that scans cannot pick up. If this has happened to you, you may well find that your idea of your baby doesn't fit with the reality, which can cause bonding issues. This does not mean you are a bad person or a bad mother. Having a newborn baby, with or without health problems, is highly stressful. It will take time for you to deal with it.

PND and traumatic birth also seem to be risk factors. (However, PND doesn't necessarily mean you won't bond with your baby – some women with PND feel passionately attached to their babies; see Chapter 2.) Kumar's study of 44 women who experienced severe bonding problems (which he dubbed 'maternal bonding disorder') found that PND and 'recalled severe pain during labour' were 'significantly' associated with their bonding difficulties. The study found no evidence that bonding difficulties are associated with a mother's character. It also found that bonding problems didn't seem limited to first babies – mothers reported having problems with a second child when they'd been fine with the first.

There is plenty of anecdotal evidence to suggest that, if you had an unhappy childhood or had a mother who herself had problems bonding with you, you may find bonding with your baby difficult – Professor Selma Frailberg's 'ghosts in the nursery' theory. There has been a lot written about 'toxic parents' who can affect an adult's relationships with their own children. If you feel that this could apply to you, see the 'Further reading' section for recommended books and websites, and have a look at Chapter 4.

Amy

My daughter was conceived through IVF, and I had a difficult pregnancy. I wanted a home birth but ended up with an emergency C-section. I then had difficulties breastfeeding and had to move on to a bottle at seven days. I think all these factors contributed to my not bonding with her.

Dawn

Two years before I got pregnant my sister's son died of cot death when he was three months old. It was an awful experience, and one of the hardest things to live with is that we don't have many photos of him. I think I didn't fully bond with my son because deep down I thought he could be taken away from me, at any time, without warning. I was very protective of him and carried a camera around with me constantly. Every time he wore a new outfit I took three photos in case the first two didn't turn out.

When my son was ten months old, my father-in-law, who lived abroad, was dying. His wife offered to pay for my partner and our son to go over for two weeks. My partner jumped at the chance, knowing his aunt was going and she'd look after our son. I was left alone and I let my hair down and went wild; I realized that I was feeling very stifled, and when my partner and son came back I told my partner I wanted to split up unless things changed.

When I saw my son at the airport, we'd been apart for two weeks but I didn't feel any emotion. I just remember thinking how unfamiliar he looked, like a stranger. When I think of this now it upsets me. It's obvious something was wrong, but at the time I hadn't been diagnosed with PND and he was my first child so I didn't know how I should feel. It was during my second pregnancy that I started to bond with my first son. He's a very mature, intelligent boy, and he was very excited about the baby.

How can I develop a bond with my baby?

There are plenty of theories flying around about how to make it more likely that you'll develop a bond with your baby. The 'attachment parenting' school of thought holds that practices such as feeding on demand, co-sleeping and carrying your baby around in a sling will help you to develop a better bond. But it's important to point out that any style of parenting that makes you and your baby happy is fine. The majority of us end up using that age-old parenting style called 'whatever works'. You don't have to call it anything or subscribe to any particular theories, or adopt an entire lifestyle if it doesn't help you – and, indeed, attempting to do this can put a great deal of pressure on you at an already very difficult time. If co-sleeping makes you happy, do it. If sleeping with your baby in another room works best for you, do it. You might like to read the 'Safer sleep advice' available on the website of the Lullaby Trust: <lullabytrust.org.uk>.

You may also be suffering from PND (see Chapter 2), which can certainly affect the quality of the maternal bond. If that's the case, your doctor may be able to offer you antidepressants or counselling. Very little research has been done on counselling to help the bonding process, but what information there is does suggest that it can be effective.

Anecdotally, it seems that time really can be a healer in some cases. It takes a while to get to know anyone, and it's far harder when that person can't even tell you what he or she likes and doesn't like, even if it is your child.

It could be that bonding is difficult simply because babies are difficult. If this is your first baby, your life will have been turned upside down. You are likely to be sleep-deprived and exhausted from breastfeeding. You could be suffering physical effects from the birth. It's normal to feel resentful, miserable or frustrated. It is also normal to be in a bad mood with your baby when he wakes up for the ninth time in a night. It's not the baby's fault, but it's easy to imagine that he or she is doing it to punish you somehow.

Things will not always be this way. Your baby will not always be a small, furious thing that does nothing but feed, sleep and excrete. As he or she grows, you will get to know the unique person that your baby is, and chances are you'll like him or her very much.

Amy, whom I interviewed for this chapter, talked about 'acting out' her feelings for her new daughter. I also tried this out and found that it helped, and it seems to be a common self-help technique among new mothers. I drew comfort from knowing that, even though I didn't feel love for him, my son would never have known it from my expressions or my actions. Habit is a powerful thing: once I fell into the habit of always waking my son up with a smile on my face, it became less of an effort. One word of warning, however: 'acting out' the feelings you'd like to have doesn't necessarily mean your true feelings go away. It's important to talk about how you feel to your partner, your health visitor or anyone else you trust. Bottling feelings up is rarely helpful because at some point they are bound to explode.

One study found that attending antenatal classes seemed to have a positive influence on maternal bonding. It could well be that being confident about looking after your baby plays a part in how well you bond with him or her.

Amy

My husband begged me to go to the doctor. I think he realized it was PND before I did and knew I needed to get some help. I had to fill in a questionnaire about how I was feeling and then the GP prescribed me some antidepressants. He also said he would call my health visitor – she has been the most amazing support for me. For days after I couldn't bring myself to do anything with my daughter, and when my husband went back to work I did what I needed to do just to get her through the day. When he came home from work he took over and I did nothing. This went on for about five weeks.

I think I started to fall in love with her when I went round to see some family with her. Of course, I had to play the 'doting mum', and while I was acting I realized that it wasn't that hard to put on the act! I realized that I liked smiling at her and talking to her and making her smile. I realized that she hadn't been hurt by how I had been to her, and because of that it was like she was giving me a second chance. I had to grab it with both hands and learn all about this new little person who was in my life.

Does it matter if we don't bond straight after birth?

It is now standard practice in the UK to put the baby to the mother's breast as soon as it is born. This is to encourage bonding and breastfeeding. In earlier decades, babies were removed, cleaned and 'topped up' with formula milk in order to give the mother a rest or to allay fears that the baby would be hungry until the mother's milk came in. It's now generally accepted that mothers and their newborns should be together in hospital to facilitate the bonding process and breastfeeding.

These first few hours are seen by some theorists as absolutely vital to developing the maternal bond. However, it's also important to remember that, if, for whatever reason, you can't spend the first few hours with your baby, this will not damage your baby in any way. Many mothers are unable to do this because they have babies who are very ill, or because they have had traumatic births that require a great deal of medical intervention. Do not feel guilty if you needed medical attention or your baby needed special care. As we've mentioned above, the bonding process is a long one. Those first few hours are important, but they're not the be-all and end-all. Thousands of babies require special care and don't get those few hours. They grow up to be just as happy and well-adjusted as the babies whose mothers were allowed to hold them.

Laura

After I had my son I only got to hold him briefly – from what I can remember it felt like a second – until I was taken down to theatre. It was about 45 minutes to an hour until I got to hold him properly. However, I did bond with him instantly. I did worry that I may not have bonded as best I could, because I feel that the minutes after a baby is born and the first time you lay eyes on the baby are when the bonding happens, and as I was in theatre my mum was left alone with him for that period of time. But my worries did not happen, and we have always been really close.

Claire

My son was induced and was born after seven hours. If I'm honest, I just felt no connection. I wanted someone to come and take him away. I didn't want him. I feel sad about feeling that about my own son. I also don't have a supportive partner, so having two children (my first daughter was two when my son was born) was a struggle in the beginning. I just got on with it.

I have an amazing friend. I rang her one day in floods of tears, and she just listened as I told her exactly how I felt. She advised me to see my GP. I didn't but I told my partner what I was feeling. It just took time, lots of it, for the cloud to slowly lift. Every day I feel guilty for the way I felt about my son. I think he knew, and that's why he was such hard work in the early months. I love my children very much, though. They are my world.

Dealing with other people's perceptions

Admitting that you do not feel love for your baby is enormously taboo and is likely to be greeted with shock. The actress Angelina Jolie attracted criticism when she described her newborn baby as a 'blob'. Even this relatively mild term – which most people who have seen a newborn will identify with – caused outrage among many parents. How could she use such a phrase to describe a gorgeous, cute, wonderful newborn baby?

Perhaps it would help mothers who find it hard to bond if society was a little more forgiving. Yes, newborn babies are miracles. But they are also hugely demanding. And it is hard to love a person who seems to do nothing but take from you, especially when you are dealing with sleep deprivation and the general uproar that a new baby – especially a first baby – brings.

Jo

My daughter was born too fast, in four and a half hours, and she tore me badly. I also needed an episiotomy and I lost too much blood. I was discharged two days later, without having my haemoglobin levels checked (no one told me about this). I went home and became ill with slurred speech which was making sense to me but not to other people. I felt faint and drunk. When my GP came out to check me and the baby a few days later, she sent me straight back to hospital as I had become severely anaemic due to so much blood loss. I had to have a blood transfusion with four pints of blood. My parents were supportive, although my dad couldn't understand why I didn't bond with my daughter, and my husband was great. I think the shock of having a blood transfusion and the shock of not knowing what to do with the baby, not being able to bond with her, caused my PND. I had never heard of it nine years ago, and no one really talked to me about it.

Will my failure to bond damage my baby?

Lack of 'maternal attachment' has been linked to everything from depression to gambling, and from addiction to eating disorders. But research in this area isn't just limited; it's extremely difficult to carry out. Most studies rely on questionnaires about the subject's childhood. Naturally, there is a pretty big margin of error. So the honest answer would be, once again, that we simply don't know. It's a given that the behaviour of a parent will affect the behaviour of a child. But it is impossible to predict how your bonding problems will affect your baby in the long term. (It's also worth noting the feminist theory that maternal attachment – or lack of it – is a male construct, a big stick to beat women with, a convenient way of blaming mothers for all their children's perceived failings. This is a pretty extreme view but when one reads of mothers being blamed for everything from obesity to unemployment, it's hard not to have some sympathy.)

But attachment, or lack of it, is just one factor in a child's development. It is interesting to note the results so far of a unique real-time study by Sir Michael Rutter's English and Romanian Adoptees Study Team into the mental health of Romanian orphans adopted by families in the West following the fall of Ceausescu in 1989. The majority of these children were found in extreme and horrific conditions that you'd imagine would scar them for life. They had no experience of any kind of parental or caregiver attachment whatsoever. However, thus far, most of them seem to be relatively well adjusted.

Hurting or neglecting your baby

In extreme cases, you may feel the urge to hurt your baby or you may not be able to care for him or her. This is rare, but it can happen. If this is the case, you need to seek help urgently from your GP, midwife, health visitor or any other health professional. If you are unable to get in touch with anyone, go to hospital. You and your baby need to have professional help as quickly as possible.

4
Family affairs

Like most thirty-something childless adults, I didn't see very much of my parents or my parents-in-law before I had my son. Sure, we met up a few times a year and got on very well. But we saw much more of our friends than we did of our family.

Of course, as soon as my son was born (indeed, before he was born), that changed. Suddenly, we found that we had a responsibility to our son's grandparents. We couldn't just tell them, as we had before, that we'd be too busy to see them for months. We had to make time for them to get to know their grandson: not easy, with both sets of parents living more than 150 miles away.

We were lucky in that both our sets of parents were supportive and helpful. But many people aren't so fortunate. Log on to any parenting website and you'll find endless stories of – in particular – mothers perceiving their mother-in-law as endlessly interfering with the upbringing of the precious new grandchild. Sometimes it's just funny, but sometimes these differences can cause real hurt to both sides. So understanding a little more about what's going on in your extended family can make it easier to head off potential conflict before it starts.

Kate

I've always had a really close relationship with both my family and my husband's family. I've known my husband since we were 15, so his family really are like 'family' to me! I get on well with his brothers and their wives, who I consider friends as well as family. Before I had children I worked for my mum and dad, and we had a good family and working relationship, and I consider my sister to be my best friend.

In my first pregnancy, I was admitted to hospital with heavy bleeding at 24 weeks, and this continued on and off until I was induced at 38 weeks. This failed, and I ended up having an emergency C-section.

My husband was away when I was first admitted, and my sister took me into hospital – she was great. My mum and dad were amazing – they wouldn't let me go back to work after that and were constantly supportive. My in-laws were OK, although they didn't seem to understand the gravity of the situation. They couldn't understand why I couldn't attend a family wedding 200 miles away when I'd just been in hospital for a week! The whole episode brought me and my husband a lot closer. He was my rock, especially while I was in hospital for the first ten days, which were the hardest.

Everything changes

It makes complete sense that your relationships with your family may change once you give birth. You have now created your own family. You've also created a new member of your extended family, and all the roles have shifted. You've gone from being sister and/or daughter to mother. Your own mother is now a grandmother. Your sisters and brothers are aunts and uncles. Your partner's family will also have these new roles to play. If your parents or parents-in-law are divorced and remarried, there will be several sets of grandparents.

Each of these roles carries different expectations and different responsibilities. Each of the people who hold these new roles will have their own ideas about the part they want to play in your new baby's life, and their perception might not square with your own.

A family time

For many women, family interference starts well before the baby is born. We have to get used to people commenting on the size of our bump, what we eat or drink, our views on childrearing and even our plans for birth. You can never predict what's coming next. My own mother-in-law was horrified when we told her we'd bought a pushchair a few months before my son was born. 'You can't have it in the house, it's bad luck!' she gasped. We pointed out that we didn't really have anywhere else to put it. (To date, we have identified no terrible events that happened because we bought a pushchair early.)

As soon as the baby is born, family members descend. I well remember attempting to entertain my mother-in-law and father-in-law after a gruelling birth and first night in hospital. If you look closely at the many pictures they took, you can just about detect the grimace beneath the smile.

It is hard enough to cope with your extended family just after a birth if you all get on. You are likely to be very tired and feeling rather helpless and disorganized, and you'll probably just want to be left alone to get to know your new baby. If, however, you don't get on with your family, then family conflict can become a real blight.

Carmel

I was about a week home from hospital when three different members of my family told me they didn't like the name we had chosen. I had no idea that the name for the baby could cause problems. I thought people would just say 'great' or 'that's lovely' even if they didn't like it. Actually, I didn't think much about other people liking it or not, so it came as a shock. Although I was confused at the time about it all, I now just think they were very rude.

My family (who are Irish) thought the name we'd chosen was really English and that it meant I was 'a traitor' calling him such a name. They also said that, if I ever moved back to Ireland with my baby, he would be teased and made fun of because of his name. My family aren't exceptionally racist, just old-fashioned, I think. I know a name might sound to some like no big deal, but it was a really big deal for me that they didn't approve and I was frightened of the baby being teased and not accepted.

I thought at the time I should change the name to please my family. It caused friction with my partner, and I was in a right muddle – as well as trying to recover from the birth and deal with sleepless nights and all the other stuff that goes with a new baby. It heightened my confusion at a very sensitive time.

In the end I discussed the matter with a psychologist who I had been seeing a few years before, and with her help I decided that the baby was having the name we had chosen and we weren't going to change it. I told my partner the baby would be named as we had first decided, and I haven't looked back (except to blow raspberries at my two brothers and my mother). My partner left me alone for a few hours one day to make up my mind – when he was gone I phoned the psychologist. When he came back, I felt I had cleared it up in my mind, definitely with the help and reassurance of the psychologist. It's all fine now, and even if they don't like the name, I don't care and it won't be changed. So far so good and no rift with my family, who seem to adore my baby, but it was such a horrible thing to do – just thoughtless I suppose.

Parenting styles

Fifty years ago formula feeding was recommended, babies routinely slept on their fronts, weaning began when you could first shove a tea-soaked rusk into your baby's mouth, and potty-training as soon as possible was the norm to avoid endless nappy bleaching and washing. It doesn't take a genius to work out how much things have changed, and of course all the advice we slavishly follow is also likely to change by the time we become grandmothers.

One of the most common complaints from new mothers is that their own mothers or mothers-in-law interfere. They criticize your chosen parenting style. They find it inexplicable that you choose to breastfeed, or to sleep in the same room or bed as your baby. After all, as the granny proclaims, you all turned out fine without this breastfeeding nonsense, or co-sleeping nonsense, or gradual weaning nonsense – so what are you worried about?

This criticism has two effects: first, you feel angry that someone else feels that he or she knows better than you, the mother; second, you feel secretly worried that perhaps you're not doing the right thing. Few first-time mothers are entirely confident in their parenting – it would be a miracle if we were. We prefer to be told that we're doing everything right.

What grandmothers say can have a huge effect on young mothers with little experience of babies. A fascinating study from Brazil examined the influence of grandmothers on breast-feeding. It found that mothers' abandoning breastfeeding in the first month was 'significantly associated' with maternal or paternal grandmothers advising them to give the baby water, tea or other milk.

How to deal with criticism

Nobody likes to be criticized, but dealing with criticism as a new mother is especially difficult. You're at your most vulnerable when you've just had a baby. Your hormones are all over the place. You are having to adjust to a completely new way of life and learn new and tricky skills like breastfeeding, all with very little sleep and possibly physical side effects following the birth. Therefore criticism or comments that previously you would have shrugged off are likely to upset you far more than usual. What you decide to do depends on so many variables – your family situation, your personality, and how often you see the person who's making the criticism.

If the criticism comes in the first few months, you may want to consider waiting until things are a little more settled before you decide what to do about it. This means gritting your teeth, bearing it and then venting to your partner afterwards, but it could potentially save you a lot of conflict.

If the criticism doesn't stop, it's time for you to consider how best to deal with it. Make sure you talk to your partner before coming up with a plan. Emphasize to them that you don't believe you're overreacting. Stay calm and don't resort to personal insults, particularly if it's their mother you're talking about. Try to decide together what you're going to do. Is it possible to sit down with the person and calmly explain to him or her that you are going to do things your way, and the criticism isn't helping? Would that make the situation worse or better? Again, avoid getting emotional. It can help to write down exactly what you want to say beforehand. Try to do it in a non-stressful situation. (It goes without saying that across the table during a family dinner is probably a bad idea.)

Ruth

I used to have a difficult relationship with my mother when I was in my twenties. When I had my first baby at 33, my mother was then 72, and although things didn't change overnight, our relationship gradually changed for the better. I think she was mellowing with age and accepting that maybe I was an adult, and I was much more sympathetic to her, partly because I was now a mother myself and partly because I made allowances for her being old. When I hear about difficult relationships between mothers, mothers-in-law and daughters, I realize how lucky I am. The perinatal time is difficult, though, because the older generation want to be seen as authorities on the subject, and the new mother sees that things have moved on, in some ways. Both my own mother and my mother-in-law made me cross by saying certain things around the childbirth–infancy stages – but that's all forgotten now. I didn't live with or anywhere near either of them, so didn't have to take any of their advice and they had no way of putting any real pressure on me to do things their way. If a new mum is not actually living with her parents or in-laws, she does not have to take any advice they give her. I remember my mum calling me 'stubborn' when I refused to give my baby a bottle. In the end you have to make your own decisions about things (it's called growing up!) and know that, whatever you do, there will be someone who'll criticize you for it. You just have to expect some criticism.

Alecia

The situation with my mother-in-law started while I was pregnant with my first son. He was not her first grandchild but her fourth. However, she was overly excited about the baby. She planned everything and bought everything she thought we needed. She didn't come to us and ask what we would like, just told us what we needed. This included pink bedding (as she said that it was a girl even though the scan showed a boy), dresses, a pushchair for a baby over six months (even though I don't drive and would need one from the time of the birth), a car seat that was for from nine months onwards (saying that babies don't need them and just put the baby in the Moses basket in the back like they did in her day), bottles (though I was very clear that I would be breastfeeding) and even a few packs of nappies, size five (they have come in handy now he is two years old).

She was so excited that she had already come up with a birth plan and decided she was going to be my birth partner (I had only met this lady after finding out I was pregnant, as her son and I met while travelling in the USA). She was very upset when I stated that her son was going to be my birth partner. She even said that the birth was more important to her than us.

After I had the baby and was still in hospital, my husband sent a text telling everyone about the baby and asking for people not to come to the hospital that day, as I had been in labour 33 hours and had had a hard time. She got very mad. I was in the hospital for

48 hours after having the baby, so I had visitors the next day. She was the first visitor and came in, picked up the baby and walked out of the room to the hall. Then, when we came home, my husband sent another text to everyone asking them to ring before coming to see the baby, as the baby and I might be sleeping. Her reply was that I was making her make an appointment before seeing her grandchild. She took everything as a rejection from me.

Then I had some family come over from overseas to see the baby. They stayed with us, and she got upset that they were there when she was to have time with the baby. My husband ended up having a fight with his mother over how she was treating me and the baby. They stopped talking. Then his whole family wouldn't talk to him, stating that he should choose his family over me and just take the baby and send me back overseas. I was still taking my son to see my family-in-law, with them saying bad things about everything I did, such as breastfeeding over a month old, not giving him chocolate right away. In the end, when my son was two and a half months old, they said they would not see my son if it was me bringing him. We have been avoiding them (as we live in the same town) ever since, and whenever I bump into them they have a go at us.

My husband has been really good through the whole thing, but it has not been easy for him. I feel bad that things have got this far, but now the situation seems to have gone on for too long and cannot be fixed. We have tried to make contact with my in-laws for our son's sake. However, we have seen from these tries that some family members are not the best people to be in our child's life.

When you dread seeing your parents

If you had an abusive childhood – or simply a difficult one – having a baby can bring all sorts of issues back into your mind that you may have managed to forget about. One of these is the prospect of seeing your parents again. It's far easier to avoid them when you don't have children. Once you have your first baby, you may feel under an obligation to include your parents, however much you may resent or fear them. This is an extra load of worry at a time when you really don't need any extra pressure. Women who experienced abuse, particularly sexual abuse, in childhood are more likely to suffer from depression. Though research in this area is limited, some studies suggest that that they are also less able to establish generational boundaries with their children and are likely to use physical punishment more frequently to discipline their children. If you feel that something in your childhood is preventing you from being the best mother you can be, think about seeking help.

We are 'supposed' to love our parents, and most of us do. But not loving a parent who has been abusive towards you is not a crime, particularly since you now have your own child to consider. You may well not want to have any contact with your parents because you want to protect your child from them. It is up to you whether you decide to carry on seeing a parent whom you cannot stand for the sake of keeping your family relationships going, or whether you decide to cut that parent out of your life altogether. These relationships are never simple, and there are, unfortunately, no easy answers. Some points to think about:

- Try to take control of the relationship. You are now an adult – you can do it. If you have agreed to meet your parents, do so at a place of your own choosing and at a time convenient for you, and limit the amount of time you spend together. Make sure your partner is there, and that they are supportive.
- Remember that, despite popular opinion, you are not destined to be your mother or your father. You are your own person. Studies have shown that many mothers from abusive families go on to be wonderful mothers themselves, sometimes through a determination to be better than their own parents.
- It may be helpful to investigate cognitive behavioural therapy techniques to help you to deal with a difficult parent. These will help you to develop ways of dealing with troubling habitual thinking and to take a more positive attitude towards yourself.
- The journey from abused child to well-balanced parent is a long and difficult one, and you may want to find out more about your options and different techniques for dealing with your past. You'll find a list of recommended books in the Further reading section.
- Bear in mind that, if it's really difficult, you don't have to see your parents at all if you don't want to or if you feel it's in

the best interests of you and your baby. Don't feel pressured by social expectations here – do what's best for you and your new family.

Lucy
What has made me saddest since having our daughter is realizing that my own childhood was not a happy time. I feel grateful to my daughter because she provided a prompt for me to seek out a counsellor and deal with some issues that had been haunting me for a long time but that I had repressed for years. This ongoing process is a painful one, but I am glad I am going through it. The insight that I am getting is improving my parenting because I'm working out exactly how I want to parent, which is completely different from how I was parented myself.

Your baby's social calendar

A friend of mine's parents are divorced and both have remarried. My friend is married to a man whose parents are also divorced and have remarried. Her baby therefore has four sets of grandparents, all of whom want to be present for baby's first Christmas. They live around 500 miles apart.

My friend's situation isn't unusual. It is now common for us to live hundreds of miles away from our parents, and the non-nuclear family is equally common. But it brings its own problems when a baby arrives – namely, who sees the baby when, and how often? For example, in-laws and your own parents can both be guilty of assuming that, now you've got a baby, they can turn up whenever they like. Being seen to spend more time with one set of grandparents than the other can also cause conflict, as can taking holidays with one set and not the other.

Again, a degree of tact is needed here, and the organizational skills of a top executive assistant wouldn't go amiss either. Here are some ideas to help you balance out the time:

- Take turns. If you spend a special occasion or religious holiday with your in-laws one year and with your own parents the next, it would be a churlish grandparent indeed who could accuse you of unfairness or favouritism. The same goes for birthdays.

- Bring grandparents together. If you think they'd get on, have them round at the same time.
- Take time off to be together as a family. It's perfectly fine to say you want to spend a weekend with no grandparents at all.
- Don't give in to unreasonable demands. You have your life, your friends, possibly your work and your baby. Your time is very precious, and it's important for you to be something other than a mother every now and again.
- Accept offers of help, but don't assume that grandparents will always be around to babysit. Perhaps they have just got work and family out of their lives, and they may well want to enjoy their newfound freedom.
- Remember that having extended family around, although it can seem like an enormous hassle, can be good for your baby and good for you. Family members provide help and 'time off' for you, they can be great alternative caregivers for your baby, and they have the priceless advantage of just being 'family' – in the best cases, people you can trust and rely on.

Katherine

I definitely got closer to my mother after having my first child. Mum and I are quite different people, but after I became a mother it seemed that we finally had something in common. Dealing with my own children has also made me appreciate how difficult parenting can be and given me a new outlook on my own childhood and my mother's parenting style. I can see now that she was working extraordinarily hard and doing her best, although at the time I took it all for granted. I've also realized that some of the things I'm most proud of as a mother are things I learned from my mum. My having a child has made a huge positive change to our relationship.

5

Baby makes three: your new relationship with your partner

For most of this chapter I am going to generally assume that your partner is male. It could well be that much of what we discuss here will apply to female partners or co-mothers as well. But all parents' experiences are different, and there is very little research on the particular challenges that co-mothers face.

I was bombarded with information and advice during my pregnancy. Leaflets and books on every aspect of birth piled up next to my bed. I spent hours on mums' forums asking about everything from the advantages of home birth to the environmental impact of disposable nappies. My husband, meanwhile, picked up one 14-page glossy magazine while waiting for me to come out of the loo at an antenatal appointment. This was the sum total of the advice given to him. The magazine dispensed pearls of wisdom for expectant dads, including top football players' comments on their babies ('It was amazing, really amazing') plus advice on not going to the pub too soon after the birth as it might annoy the wife. Not exactly comprehensive.

After an amusing session sneering at the 'tips', which seemed to have been written on the assumption that men know rather less about birth than your average goldfish, we both felt rather depressed. It's hardly surprising that, with information being as scarce as this, the birth of a baby becomes, for the partner, a rather mysterious and frightening event to be left to the women – shades of the olden days when men were bundled out of the house while the midwife rolled up her sleeves and took over the messy, embarrassing part, and the grandmother was there to do the nappy changing for the first month.

Having a baby is a defining moment in a relationship, in many cases far more so than getting married or moving in together. It's a lot easier to divorce someone than it is to split up a family, and it's a lot easier to just move yourself out. A baby is a different kind of commitment. A baby has no choice in the matter. A baby is a tangible product of your relationship. And having a baby can be very, very hard.

The practical impact of a baby on your relationship with your partner is easy to quantify. It's fairly obvious that broken nights, breastfeeding, lack of sex and loss of former free time will lead to one or both of you being more irritable than usual. The emotional impact is less easy to measure. Birth, as we have already mentioned, can bring up a lot of negative and unfamiliar feelings – in partners as well as mothers. Jealousy, feelings of inferiority, fear, loss of control, loss of libido – all of these are common in those difficult first few months. If you have PND or have been traumatized by the birth of your child, your partner may well need to support both of you.

There is also a growing body of evidence suggesting that male partners may also be susceptible to PND, and that they can also experience PTSD after witnessing a traumatic birth. And more men are speaking out: Mark Williams founded the UK charity Fathers Reaching Out after experiencing panic attacks and postnatal depression following the traumatic birth of his son and his wife Michelle's severe PND. One US study found that 14 per cent of mothers and 10 per cent of fathers exhibited levels of depressive symptoms.

And, of course, not all partners are male. How a traumatic birth or a new mother suffering from PND might affect their female partner is an area that deserves much more attention. One small-scale review carried out by antenatal practitioner Katherine Walker points out that, just as for male partners, 'much of the work for a lesbian co-mother (LCM) is emotional adaptation rather than physical recovery' following the birth. She highlights the fact that lack of support is a trigger for PND, and that co-mothers may be at greater risk if their family relationships are strained.

Again, it is important to stress that if you are that partner – male or female – you are not alone, and your feelings are valid. Do not ever be afraid of seeking help because you were not the one who gave birth.

Is my relationship at risk?

It's impossible to predict how your relationship will be affected by your baby. However, studies have shown that certain risk factors (discussed below) make the likelihood of a rocky road more common, although, of course, you may not fall into any of these categories and still have difficulties at this time, which one study refers to as a 'psychosocial trauma'.

A volatile relationship

Throughout the ages, married couples have had babies to try to salvage a troubled relationship. It's only recently that someone's given this a catchy name – a 'sticking-plaster baby'. One study followed 43 couples who became parents. They were interviewed about the relationship when they got married. What predicted the stable or increasing marital satisfaction of mothers were the husband's expressions of fondness towards her, the husband's high regard for her and their relationship, and her regard for her husband and their relationship. In contrast, what predicted the decline in marital satisfaction of mothers were the husband's negativity towards his wife, the husband's disappointment in the marriage, or the husband or wife having described their lives as chaotic.

It seems obvious, but it is worth pointing out, that if you didn't have a great relationship before your baby arrived, you are less likely to have a brilliant one now that you have all the added pressures of parenthood. Another study from the Netherlands found that the more conflict there is generally in your relationship, the more conflict you are likely to experience during the transition to parenthood.

An unplanned pregnancy

We are so used to controlling every aspect of our lives these days that it can be a huge shock when, for example, contraception doesn't work. Although many couples can (and do) come to terms with the shock of an unplanned pregnancy as it progresses, research has shown that the fathers of unplanned babies do find it much harder to get to know and love their children. A study from the University of Washington that analysed levels of marital satisfaction after the birth of a first baby found that couples who had had a planned pregnancy had higher 'satisfaction scores'.

A non-mutual decision

If your partner didn't want you to get pregnant, they will find it harder to cope. Of course, it's natural for both of you to feel ambivalent about your decision at times. But that's a very different feeling from the clearly stated desire not to have a baby at all. A study published in the *Journal of Marriage and Family* found that men who didn't want their partners to get pregnant were less likely to show 'parental warmth' towards their new babies.

How your relationship changes

Before the baby arrives, the majority of couples don't have to negotiate who works on what days, or who goes to the gym in the evening. Your time is, very broadly speaking, your own. Then the baby arrives – and suddenly, things are very different. The mother is, still, usually the one who takes the most leave, despite shared parental leave becoming more common. And it is still the case that women are more likely to give up their jobs once they have a baby, although research suggests that the number of 'stay-at-home' dads is on the rise.

It's a dramatic shift in roles and one that can cause a great deal of conflict and change, usually around two areas: the division of labour and the woman's change of role from that of lover to that of mother.

Carmel

My partner didn't realize how much I was in need of some rest and looking after. He was so excited by the birth that he actually wasn't much help to me – he became hyperactive and was on cloud nine, on another planet. He had hardly any sleep for a couple of nights during the labour either, and then the night after Ryan was born, he got completely drunk with his friend and stayed up all night again. He arrived at the hospital the next day, and when I came back from the toilet, he was asleep – in the same clothes from the day before, unshaven and smelling of alcohol – on my hospital bed. At that moment, I felt things really weren't right, and although overjoyed with the baby, I was struggling to cope with the exhaustion. The idea was that I could get some sleep while my partner looked after the baby for a few hours, but that nevver happened in the hospital, and the midwives were too busy to help me out either.

I started to feel better once I got home, but I never really caught up on the sleep lost. And as my partner is very extrovert, he kept insisting we have visitors almost every day to show them the new baby, which left me even more drained. I think that, all this time, I wasn't confident enough to put my foot down enough with him, and I ended up feeling like I never wanted a guest again. While having Ryan was the best thing ever, I felt stressed and extremely tired and was crabby with my partner at this time. When you have a new baby, a lot of people don't want to hear you complain as it doesn't fit their ideals – they can also get the wrong end of the stick very easily and think you don't want the baby! As my partner is a stimulation junkie, he didn't really get it when I told him I wanted peace and quiet to recover from the birth and sleep loss.

I can look back at this now and I see that I should have been firm and unapologetic about what my limits were so that I could have coped better. That is actually what I have done the past few months and I am all the better for it. Things are great with my partner now too, and I'm not annoyed with him like I used to be. His extra energy is actually really useful at times, and he is helpful around the house and an excellent dad. Also, he does get it now that I have limits.

Division of labour

A recent study found that women in couples do, on average, 15 hours a week of housework, while men in partnerships do five hours. There is a common idea, particularly among men, that being at home with a baby all day is some kind of rest cure. This, as you no doubt already know, is not the case. There is washing, cleaning, feeding, nappy changing and more feeding to be done – all while you are tired and your baby is demanding your attention. Being at home with the baby does not therefore mean that you have plenty of time to do the usual household chores. You may have to point this out to your partner. Remember, neither of you has had a baby before. They may really think that you're living a life of leisure.

If they are expecting more of you than you can give, it's time to do some straight talking. Yes, they are at work all day, but so are you – and you don't get to clock off at half past five. Draw up a list of things that have to be done and divide them evenly between you. Learn to overlook things – does it really matter that the front room now gets vacuumed once a week rather than three times? Above all, make it clear that your new relationship is still one of equals. If you want to take on extra chores around the house, that's fine – just make sure it's your decision. Don't feel forced or emotionally blackmailed into doing more. You only have room for one child in the house now.

Lucy
It's surprised me how well my husband and I work as a team in terms of our baby's care; somehow I expected to feel much more put upon, but he pulls his weight and is happy to do so. That makes a big difference. We are also lucky to have his mum around, who helps out.

Lover to mother

Birth means you have gone through huge physical and mental changes. And your partner's life will change too. But these changes will be slower and less obvious. I will never forget the words of one woman who posted on a parenting website about her husband's attempt at making her understand how he felt. He wished that things could be the way they were, that he could have his 'old life' back with all the freedom that entailed. Her response was to snap, 'Well, I wish I could wee without painkillers.'

A 2018 study of 832 first-time mothers found that nearly half of them reported a lack of interest in sexual activity. It found that 43 per cent suffered from vaginal dryness and 37.5 per cent were still finding sex difficult or painful six months after the birth. This was associated with having had a vacuum-assisted birth, a second- or, third-degree perineal tear or an episiotomy. Breastfeeding was also cited as a major factor associated with a lack of interest in sex, as was a feeling of dissatisfaction with their body's appearance.

A small study of Thai women in 2007 found the 'influencing factor' in resuming a sex life after having given birth was 'the sexual demand of the partner'. If the birth was traumatic, it may be a long time before you feel mentally able to have sex again. Physical trauma can also mean no sex, as can lack of sleep, lack of privacy and lack of time, all of which lead to lack of libido. Some women who have suffered birth trauma also find that sex is difficult because it's connected to a fear of getting pregnant again. And body issues can also play a part: a study from the University of Virginia found that 12 months after the birth of a first child, both mothers and fathers still had concerns around how they or their partner looked.

Nicola
I was obsessive about using contraception because I couldn't bear the thought of having another child.

There are no concrete guidelines stating when it's 'normal' to have sex again after giving birth – how you feel is the best indicator. If you've had an episiotomy or a Caesarean delivery, it's wise to wait until you've healed. Likewise, there is no set amount of sex you should be aiming for. Sex surveys are not particularly reliable sources of information but they can provide something of a blurry snapshot. A survey of 20,000 UK parents by BabyCentre, an online resource for expectant and new mothers, found that most parents had sex around three to five times a month six months after the birth of their child. So don't be under the impression that everyone else is having sex six times a day, hanging off the ceiling. It simply isn't true. Take as much time as you need.

It may be that your partner wants sex before you feel ready. Talking about how you feel is vital. If you don't feel ready for sex, tell them honestly. Nobody has the right to demand sex from you if you don't want to do it. Don't go through with it just to keep them happy – that's not good for either of you.

You should remember, too, that intimacy and closeness don't always mean sex. Cuddling, touching and foreplay will help you rediscover your sexual selves and allow you some time to be partners, not parents. 'Scheduling' sex might sound rather horrendous but, if possible, try to have time together while your baby's asleep. Try to keep this part of your relationship alive as you go through this stressful time.

If you are still finding the idea of sex very distressing or you find having sex painful after the birth, talk about it to your health visitor, practice nurse or doctor. Physical and mental problems with sex after birth can be treated and they are very common – one study found that, out of 484 respondent women, 83 per cent had experienced sexual problems up to three months after their babies were born. Try to get advice as soon as you realize that something's wrong.

(Incidentally, I was advised to have sex before my routine six-week check-up to see whether there were any medical issues. I accepted this advice without question. In retrospect, I should have said that I would have sex when I was ready, and not before.)

Why do some partners find it hard to bond with their babies?

It can be hard to feel involved with a pregnancy if you are not the pregnant one. The prospective mother is carrying the child. She is the one who has to put up with the backache, the nausea, the exhaustion and the eight-times-a-night trips to the toilet, and all those niggling annoyances which occur during even the easiest pregnancy. She gets the first kick, the first hiccup, the feeling of achievement that she is creating something new and wonderful. She is the one getting all the congratulations and all the attention. Consequently, the baby can seem more 'real' to her. Her involvement with her baby begins far sooner than her partner's. She generally finds it easier to think about the future with a baby.

After the baby is born, all the advice and help will, again, be concentrated on the mother. Breastfeeding is something only she can do. She may appear more tuned into the baby's needs. She may respond more quickly to her baby's crying. She may only have eyes for her baby and think and talk about nothing else. She may be unwilling to let other people look after her baby. In short, all her attention will probably be focused on her baby and not on her partner. This is, of course, completely normal. But it can be very hard for partners to comprehend.

I've heard many partners say that they feel shut out from their babies. It's not quite the same as jealousy. They want to bond, they want to get to know their children – but they don't know how. As I mentioned previously, it's unsurprising that partners are nervous when the baby comes home – they haven't got a clue what to do. Quite a few mothers also feel this way. (I informed my husband on the day we brought our son home that the possession of a vagina does not confer magical baby skills.) But at least we're more likely to have attended antenatal classes or to have been shown what to do by a midwife or nurse. Also, we've usually already had a day or two of looking after our baby in hospital. So we get a head start in all these new skills – nappy changing, bathing, feeding, holding, and working out how the poppers go together in the crotch of sleep-suits.

Your partner may well want to help, and if you want them to help for the next 18 years it's a good idea to get them involved at the start. You may be slightly irrational about their involvement. They may bathe the baby in a different way. They may, on their first few tries, do the nappy up incorrectly. However, these minor mistakes do not mean that your partner is a fool incapable of doing the simplest thing for your child. It's important that you allow them to make mistakes and deal with the consequences. They will very soon discover that doing a nappy up incorrectly means they will spend the next hour cleaning poo off the Moses basket. This is a great learning experience. They are unlikely to put the nappy on the wrong way again.

This sounds light-hearted, but there is a serious side to it. At some point, you will want to reclaim some aspects of your former life. You'll want to go out and see your friends. If you can't leave your baby with your partner because they don't know how to look after their child, you are in for serious problems. You'll wonder why they are so useless, why they claim they can't do the simplest thing. So let go of the reins a bit. It's hard when you're a first-time mother and you're convinced that you do everything far better than them. But allowing them to get used to the daily routine of childcare will make things far easier for you as a couple further down the line. Give your partner that responsibility.

You'll also be giving your partner a great gift: that of getting to know your child. You don't get to know a baby just by being there at the cute moments. It's a relationship that starts with the very basics – being there to clean and feed him or her. Don't shut your partner out of this amazing process.

The above also holds true for partners who may appear completely uninterested or say they don't 'do' babies. It's a learning and a getting-to-know-you process for all three of you. Encourage your partner to get involved and you should find after a while that they want to be involved.

Jealous partners

There are two schools of thought on partner jealousy. One runs something like this: any adult who is jealous of a tiny baby has something very wrong with them and should be told to get over themselves. The other runs something like this: it may seem to be irrational to be jealous of one's own son or daughter, but it actually makes perfect sense. If you've previously been the centre of someone's life, it's natural to feel jealous when one day she suddenly dedicates every waking moment to someone else – particularly when that someone else is a constantly screaming baby. Therefore it might help to understand why a partner might feel jealous and to work together to solve the problem.

How do you know your partner is jealous? Listen to what they tell you. Jokey comments such as 'You love that baby more than me', 'You've never tucked me up in bed / given me a bath / given me a massage' or 'I never see you alone these days' could all indicate that they are feeling left out and envious of the attention you give to your baby. Some partners may come right out and say it. Some will bottle it up and express their jealousy in other ways, usually by disappearing for hours on end or throwing themselves into their work. A few will be actively hostile towards their baby.

Jealousy can poison a relationship – any relationship. If you think your partner is jealous, try to get them to talk about it. In an ideal world, you should not have to bear this burden on top of being a first-time mother. However, if you can offer your partner a listening ear, you may find that they are a lot more help to you in the future. A little attention at this crucial point can pay off. This isn't about mothering, enabling or indulging your partner – it's about taking the issue seriously.

Finding the right time and place to talk is vital. Don't bring up any of these issues during stressful times, while the baby is crying or when you're trying to feed or change him or her. Sort out some baby-free time. For example, go for a walk – your baby will, you can hope, fall asleep in the buggy or pram and you can talk and walk at the same time. If your baby naps at set times, aim for one of those as your talking time. Or, if your baby is old enough and you feel comfortable leaving him or her, try to get a trusted friend or relative to babysit for an hour or so. That's long enough for you and your partner to go and have a coffee somewhere baby-free.

Try not to be too accusatory. Reassure your partner that what they are feeling is normal. Point out to them that this is the time when your baby needs his mother most – literally so if you're breastfeeding. It won't be like this for the rest of your lives. It's very hard to see beyond the first hundred crazy days of your baby's life (a friend of mine calls them 'the hundred days of hell', a description I enthusiastically adopted). Remind your partner that in just a few months your son or daughter will be smiling, crawling, talking and openly expressing love – the baby won't always be a squalling, red-faced poo machine. And encourage your partner to do things with the baby. If you are bottle-feeding or expressing, get your partner to do one feed a day – perhaps a night feed, so you can have a break. If you're breastfeeding exclusively, make these times togetherness times as a family. Allow them to take responsibility and let them spend time on their own with the baby, so they can develop their relationship.

Niamh

I was aware that 'baby blues' were normal, but my feelings of sadness seemed to linger months after her birth. My husband (now ex-husband!) had a 'get up and on with it' attitude. I didn't seek any medical attention at this stage. I didn't talk to anyone because 17 years ago depression was not as accepted as it is now. I didn't get much support from my husband, so I figured nobody else would understand if he didn't.

Jealous mothers

A problem that receives rather less attention is that of the mother who feels her baby loves her partner more than her. This often, but not always, goes hand in hand with PND and bonding issues.

I have personal experience of this. It was my husband who held our son properly for the first time, and it was my husband who held his hand while he had his vitamin K injection and was checked over. Later, it was my husband who looked after our boy as he had numerous blood tests and check-ups. I was in too much of a state to do anything. I realized that my husband had formed a special bond with my son, and I was gutted rather than happy that my partner had adjusted to fatherhood so well. I thought that it should have been me. I had heard so much about the fabled mother–baby bond and partner jealousy that it never occurred to me that I might be the one with envy issues.

Here, again, it's important to talk to your partner. Let them know how you are feeling. These are complex emotions, easily misunderstood and not easily put into words. A talk with good intentions can easily break down into an accusing session. It might help to write down what you want to say before you say it, to make sure you know exactly what you want to convey. Again, try to talk in a non-stressful setting. Try to spend time alone with your baby. Relationships don't just develop out of nowhere. They have to be worked on. It can be the same with babies. Remember that your partner is not trying to get one over on you – it's not a competition to see which parent your baby loves the most. Chances are that your partner will be expecting you to be pleased that they love their new child so much, and it may be a rude awakening when they realize it's not the case.

Amy
I started watching how my husband was with the baby, and then when I was alone I tried doing it myself. It did feel odd at first as all I could think of was how awful I had been to her. But she reacted back to me and started doing more each day. She developed her own little personality, and I started to learn her likes and dislikes.

Counselling for couples

Many couples find that conflict lessens over time as they both settle into their new roles. But if you are having real problems communicating a few months down the line, it may be worth considering couples' counselling, available from organizations such as Relate (see 'Useful contacts' for details). It can be very useful to have an outsider's perspective on your relationship. Counselling can help you to communicate again and can have great results.

Moving on

Yes, the first few months of your baby's life are one of the most testing times for a couple, but they can be one of the more rewarding ones as well. Having a baby is a true act of partnership. You brought this baby into the world together, and you can bring it up together too. When you and your partner work as a team, parenthood becomes a joyful, enriching experience. It enhances your relationship. You see sides of your partner you have never seen before, and you learn more about your partner than you ever expected.

A 2008 Swedish study examined the experiences of 20 first-time fathers who were aged between 20 and 48. The main theme that emerged was, unsurprisingly, 'changing life'. But those changes seemed to be mainly positive. Fathers discussed how 'wonderful' they found fatherhood and how, although their relationship with their partner had changed, those changes were usually for the better.

Laura
Our relationship got better after our little one was born. Before he was born we used to argue a lot more. When he arrived things changed. Our priorities changed, and he was our most important thing. I suffered birth trauma and PND, but my partner was a superstar. He hardly ever did any housework before, but after the baby was born that was it, he was doing everything. He made me rest and told me just to focus on our son. I did do things but knew that, if I didn't have time, then I could rely on him. We bonded so much and he loved my body even more because it had carried our son. We stuck together through this. We decided we would tackle the problem as a team and reminded ourselves of our love.

6
Adjusting to a new you

During your pregnancy, you may have encountered various Cassandras who say unhelpful things such as 'Well, say goodbye to ever finishing a book, or watching a film, or going hiking.' While there may be some truth in this, it is certainly not the whole truth of motherhood, and it's this kind of attitude that makes many of us fearful that, once we give birth, our lives and our personalities will be lost beneath a great wave of nappies and baby food.

Becoming a mother does change you, but not in the ways you might expect. Your body will change. Your relationships with your partner and family are likely to change. You may find you look at various issues differently now you have a baby. But ultimately you are still the same person that you were. You don't suddenly become a saint. You don't have a personality transplant along with the epidural. If you were impatient before, chances are you'll still be impatient.

Lucy
Becoming a mother has changed everything and nothing about me. I still enjoy my marriage, my work, my hobbies, my friends and nights out, but the parameters are different. I work three days a week instead of five or six; nights out are rare and I see much less of friends (especially those friends who don't have kids!). I did not expect parenthood to be as rewarding as it is and yet also so tedious! I swell with pride in the evenings when my husband and I talk about our daughter's latest milestones, something funny that's she's done or something that made her laugh. And yet I get wound up when she won't open her mouth for me to clean her teeth, chucks yogurt on the floor, or refuses to put her coat and shoes on to go out. It never ceases to amaze me how you can feel so many different emotions in one day when you're with your child. When I compare that with how life was before, it's like the difference between a mobile phone and a smartphone.

How having a baby changes your body

I remember looking down at my stomach just after giving birth and being surprised that I still looked pregnant. This is how much I knew about what your body does after birth. Three months later, I still looked pregnant. In purely physical terms, this is how your body changes. You are likely to have put on several stone. Quite a lot of this is baby but some of it isn't – after all, few of us bother counting calories during pregnancy. In the last few months of pregnancy, the majority of mothers don't take strenuous exercise. We are simply too exhausted. You might also have a condition that limits your movement, such as symphysis pubis dysfunction (SPD), and makes exercise very difficult or impossible.

Your bump will have stretched the skin on your stomach, so it's likely to feel and look loose and floppy. You're unlikely to have got your waistline back. Your breasts will probably be larger and feel more floppy, although they may return to their pre-pregnancy size when you stop breastfeeding. You may have swollen ankles and stretch marks on your stomach, thighs or breasts. You may feel that your vagina isn't as 'tight' as it was before.

All these changes are natural and normal, but they can take a lot of getting used to. It's a very strange feeling looking down at your body and not recognizing it as your own, although it's one you may well have felt when your bump first started to appear.

Celebrity pressures

A 2014 report for the Government Equalities Office highlighted that the constant bombardment from media images lauding celebrity mothers who 'snap back' into size 8 jeans just a few weeks after giving birth can be hugely damaging. Authors Susie Orbach and Holli Rubin write that these images are 'switching the focus of the post-partum period away from mother and baby getting to know each other and finding a rhythm together. Instead there is a cultural insinuation that a mother's job is to present herself physically as though nothing as momentously life-changing or body-changing as having a baby has occurred. This critical moment, in which new life and the new mother weave together a delicate and precious bond, needs supporting in order to ensure the best possibilities for both.'

It's worth saying again and again: celebrities are not realistic role models. If you have a full-time day nanny, a night nanny, a personal trainer, a chef, a stylist and your own in-house gym, you're allowed to compare yourself to a celebrity. If, like most of us, you don't, then relax. You have far more important things to worry about than the size of Kim Kardashian's waist compared with yours.

This isn't to devalue looking good. Taking care of yourself is important in this time of change. It can be a way of doing something for yourself, clawing back a little bit of your day for you and you alone. If putting on body lotion and shaving your legs and doing your hair was important to you before you got pregnant, it's likely to be important to you afterwards. (Or you may feel perfectly justified in happily slobbing around in pyjamas all day – in which case, good for you.) The important factor in self-image after you give birth is doing what makes you feel good for you, not for your partner and not for some celebrity yardstick.

Safe weight loss

It takes nine months to grow a baby, and the prevailing wisdom is that it takes another nine months for your body to return to normal. Everyone's different. Some women find that they lose weight naturally and quickly. Others find it harder to shift the weight. One Australian study found that dissatisfaction with your body seems to peak at around six months after you give birth; perhaps this is when things start to settle down and you've actually got time to think about losing weight.

Not much research has been carried out on the best ways to lose your baby weight, although there are thousands of people out there claiming they have the way. Be wary of fad diets and exercise programmes. In terms of exercise, think about doing what you enjoy – if you try to stick to an impossible gym programme when you hate the gym and you can't leave your baby anyway, you're setting yourself up for failure. A 2014 review of the available literature found that the most effective way of losing baby weight seemed to be a combination of sensible diet and exercise, so try to mix the two.

When can I exercise again?

This depends on an awful lot of variables – how fit you were before and during your pregnancy, the kind of birth you had and simply how you feel. We've all heard stories about athletes who were back on the treadmill within a week, but that's not the experience of most women. Most doctors will recommend waiting around six weeks before you start exercising again. This is to allow time for the uterus to contract and go back to its usual size and for joints and pelvic ligaments, which have been loosened by pregnancy, to return to normal.

In the meantime, however, make sure you still get out and about. Exercise has been linked to improved mood among patients with depression, and going out for a walk is good for your head as well as your body. Get back on your bike if you used to cycle before you got pregnant. It's also worth looking out for a postnatal exercise class where you can take your baby. Make sure you get the all-clear from your doctor before you resume any kind of exercise programme in the first couple of months following the birth, particularly if it's something you're new to or if it's something that involves putting a lot of strain on your abdomen.

When is it safe for me to diet again?

If you are breastfeeding, talk to your doctor or midwife before you start any kind of diet. It's generally recommended that you shouldn't start a diet when breastfeeding, since you need extra calories to make the milk and to stay healthy and energized yourself. However, some women find that breastfeeding helps them lose the weight they've gained in pregnancy.

You may not need to diet at all – just take your time, eat a healthy balanced diet and stay active. A healthy balanced diet is one that doesn't go overboard on fatty and sugary foods, and contains a wide variety within all the major food groups:

- rice, potatoes, pasta and other starchy foods
- fruit and vegetables

- milk and other dairy foods
- meat, fish, eggs, beans and other non-dairy sources of protein.

If you do decide to go on a diet, avoid fad diets since these are not good at helping you lose weight in the long term. Forming good eating and exercise habits is the key to healthy weight loss. Don't be downhearted at tales of other women fitting into size 8 jeans a week after they've given birth. Everyone's metabolism is different. As a new mother, you're under enough pressure just keeping things together. Try not to let your weight become an issue.

Coming to terms with your new body

Becoming a mother is about accepting change and realizing that things are never going to be the way they were. That's not necessarily a bad thing, and it applies to your body as well. You can try to pretend the birth didn't happen and spend the next three years trying to eradicate stretch marks, saving up for boob jobs and tummy tucks, spending six hours a week on a treadmill or eating nothing but tofu. Cosmetic science has given us ways of turning back the clock, for a price. It's foolish to pretend that these options don't exist. Perhaps they might work for you. But really, they're only delaying the inevitable – after all, your body will change as it gets older and, unless you're Madonna, there's not much you can do about that. The changes motherhood brings to your body are a part of life.

I've heard women justify cosmetic surgery after childbirth as a way of 'feeling good about themselves'. If you need drastic surgery performed under anaesthetic in order to feel good about yourself after giving birth, you may well have some underlying issues about becoming a mother that you haven't resolved. There are easier, safer and cheaper ways to feel good about yourself, and chief among these is improving your self-image. Your mind needs work before your body does. Try the following ways of coming to terms with your new shape:

- Don't buy clothes a size smaller in the hope that you'll fit into them or hang on to pre-pregnancy jeans. You're only setting yourself up for a disappointment. Instead, why not buy some cheap clothes a size larger than you would normally need? They'll do you fine until you're ready to think about whether you want to lose weight or not.

- Don't compare yourself to other women. Everyone is different. Celebrities are not realistic role models.
- Do things that aren't about how your body looks but how it feels. Get your partner to look after the baby while you have a bath and wallow in bubbles. Treat yourself to a nice body lotion. Go to the hairdresser's or have a massage.
- If your body shape has changed a lot, book a personal shopper consultation to find the clothes that look great for your new body shape – most major department stores now offer this service.
- Get yourself measured when you go and buy a new bra. Thousands of women are wearing the wrong bra size, and you'll be amazed at how much better your breasts feel and look when they're in a bra that's the correct size for you.
- When your partner tells you that they still fancy you and you look great, believe them.
- Think more about what your body can do, not what it looks like. You grew and nurtured your child for nine months. Now it's your body, your skin and your smell that calm your baby and make him or her feel secure and needed. That's an amazing thing.

Joanne
I felt much more positive about my body after having children. I had always thought that my life would be much better if I weighed less and was better looking. Suddenly I realized that my body was this amazing instrument that could nurture and produce life. I don't mind things like stretch marks because I believe that your body is a map of your life, and they're a badge of honour. I could do without the wobbly tum and random lumps and bumps, but hey-ho, it's just part of the process, isn't it?

Playing mother

In the early days of motherhood I felt very much as if I was playing a part, and I wasn't quite sure of the lines, or where I should be standing, or indeed whether or not I should have been picked to play the role at all. I still feel like that sometimes. Perhaps everyone does, but few admit it.

The word 'mother' has, as we've discussed, certain connotations: saintly, wise, patient, fount of all wisdom and joy, and so on. And, for some reason, we continue to hold on to these traditional mother stereotypes and then beat ourselves up if we don't conform to them. 'She's a natural mother,' people say when watching a new mum with her baby. Yet is there really any such thing? It could simply be that some of us adjust better to being mothers than others. That's very different from the idea that we all have some 'natural', inbuilt tendency to be a 'good mother'. I'm not talking about the ability to feed and change a child – anyone can learn this. I'm talking about those other feelings – about how you feel about being a mother rather than the acts of mothering.

The fact is that many of us don't particularly like 'being a mother' for the first few months. We may resent the huge impact a child has had on our lives. We hate the sleepless nights, the endless round of feeding and nappy changing. And then we berate ourselves because we don't conform to the popular stereotype – and that must mean that we're 'bad mothers', surely?

It has never been easier to believe that you're a 'bad mother'. There have never been so many rules to be broken unwittingly, never so many tiny points of parenting etiquette to be accidentally flouted, never so many books containing precisely opposing childrearing techniques, never so many social problems that are the 'fault of the parents' (in other words, the mother). Never before has an uncertain mother had the facility to stick her problem on a parenting website forum and instantly find 50 people she's never met denouncing her. Perhaps there's something to be said for the mother-in-law who mutters about how in her day you just got on with it and asked Granny.

For some reason, women who previously would never have fallen for easy societal stereotypes start worrying once they become mothers. The image of motherhood is so old, so pervasive and so ingrained in every aspect of our culture that it's not difficult to see why. We start measuring ourselves against impossible role models. We think back to our mothers and grandmothers who seemed to devote every moment of their lives to their children. Are we wrong to want to keep our identities? I don't think so. It is possible to be a mother and to be yourself as well.

> *Cath*
> I'm suffering from PND at the moment, and I'm sure that the sudden and massive focus upon my becoming a mother by everyone around me hasn't helped at all. Perhaps it's because I don't like to be pigeon-holed, but everyone seems to have forgotten that I'm also a journalist, a runner, a gardener … The upshot is that I never seem to get a break from being a mother. Babies are the only topic of conversation among many of my friends and family now, and I can't stand that. There is so much more going on in my mind and my life other than dirty nappies and night feeds! It's why I'm still taking on work. It's exhausting, but at least it's a touch of normality and reminds me that life is about more than cooing at a mewling child.
>
> Everyone says the same old, same old to me – that I must be madly in love with my baby, that I probably can't remember what life was like before she came, that I wouldn't swap her for anything now. But the truth is that I don't feel any of these things, so I feel as if I'm missing something that everyone else has experienced. The only time I don't feel as if I'm failing is when none of these expectations is placed upon me. People are well meaning but blind to the fact that motherhood comes in all shapes and forms. I don't fit that glowing, maternal, beatific mould, and having that image foisted upon me all the time is an enormous strain when I'm already all too aware of how I'm struggling.

There's nothing wrong with wanting to carry on doing the things you love. You may have to change the way you do them or who you do them with, or do them less frequently. But don't feel that you have to drop your karate class, for example, or your book club, or your weekend away with the girls, just because you're now a mother. These are the things that make you 'you'. Holding on to these things will require a bit of extra effort, but it's worth it to retain your sense of self.

Negotiate with your partner to get the time you need. From the beginning, it helps to make it very clear that being a mother is a full-time job in itself and you will need some time off. It's equally important that your partner can carry on doing the things that they enjoy, so decide between yourselves who's going to do what and when. You might both have to compromise, but that's what an equal partnership is all about.

Joanne

I can't bear being called 'Mummy', other than by my kids. It feels so dismissive, like you're just defined by the fact that you have children and nothing else. Chuggers are the worst for doing this – I am normally quite a calm person, but there's something about an 18-year-old saying 'Hello, Mum' that makes me want to punch them. Usually I ignore them, but recently when one chugger came at me with a 'Hi, Mum!' I snapped back with 'I'm not your mum, don't be so patronizing.' But he wasn't offended – still kept smiling! That made me want to belt him even more.

Babies and friends

Once you have a baby, you are likely to see your childless friends less. That doesn't mean you'll lose them – it's a simple matter of practicality. Once you have a baby, you'll probably find that you need to plan ahead more. It will no longer be practical for people to just turn up for a quick drink since you'll be putting your baby to bed. You may not be able to accept spur-of-the-moment invitations since you'll need time to organize babysitting or else have your partner come home early. I often think they should add a couple of new time zones – 'Baby Time' and 'No-Baby Time'. Living on Baby Time involves getting up at 6 a.m., being up in the night, having to stop everything to feed five times a day and collapsing on the sofa at around 7 p.m. if you're lucky, hoping for a few hours of me-time before the crying starts again. Living on No-Baby Time involves doing basically what you like when you like.

Don't expect friends to know this automatically. Until you're in the eye of the storm, it's very hard to appreciate how Baby Time can completely take over your life. Some people will realize that your schedule has altered and will be considerate, some will not. Some people may need a bit of gentle re-education. It may be that you will lose contact with some of your childless friends. It's always a shame when friends grow apart, but this is natural. Rest assured that you will find new ones.

Enjoying your new role

If you're lonely and don't have any support from friends and family, you're more likely to suffer from PND. So start building your support networks. If you've suffered or are still suffering from PND or PTSD, doing this can be very challenging. Not every mother enjoys baby-and-toddler groups, and not everyone has attended antenatal classes where you can get to know other mothers-to-be before you give birth. If you have family around to lend a hand, that's fantastic, but you can't expect family members to offer help or company as a given – many grand-mothers these days lead just as busy and fulfilling lives as their daughters and can't always be called upon at the drop of a hat. And, in any case, some grandmothers may simply not want to look after a baby.

Start small. Remember, you're not looking for a best friend here (although, if you find one, that's great). You're looking for people like you who have small babies and would just like someone to pass the time of day with – going to the park for the fifth time in a week is so much more fun when you've got adult company. Try the following ideas:

- Ask your health visitor if anyone else has recently given birth in your immediate area and, if so, whether he or she would be willing to sound her out about meeting up. You never know – you may find someone just down the road from you.
- Give baby-and-toddler groups a try. You may have a great time, you may not, but it's worth a go. Groups that are run or supervised by a health visitor tend to be less intimidating than informally run groups – the supervisor will make sure you feel included, especially if you let him or her know beforehand if you have PND.
- See what classes are available in your area, such as baby swimming, baby massage, baby yoga or baby music, or movement classes like Tumble Tots. These are a good way to get out of the house if you have PND. Everyone is focused on the activity, so it won't matter if you don't feel like making conversation. The activity itself gives everyone something to talk about. An activity that happens at the same time each

week means that you can start to build a routine, which can really help you get your sense of 'real life' back. Ask your health visitor or midwife about what's available in your area.

- Look on parenting forums and apps to see whether there are any other new mothers in your area. If you are meeting someone you've contacted online for the first time, ensure that you take sensible precautions. Don't give out any personal information online or at your first meeting, always meet initially in a public place such as a café or soft play centre, make sure you let someone else know where you're going, and trust your instincts – if something (or someone) 'feels' wrong, it probably is wrong.

Going back to work or not

Whether or when to go back to work is one of the most difficult areas to deal with when you become a mother. What you decide to do about work will depend on your financial situation, your personal situation (for example, if you are a single mother you may have no choice about whether or not to work) and quite simply how you feel about being a working mother. Some women decide to give up work and become full-time mothers. Some decide to go back to work full-time or part-time. Some decide to go in a different direction and retrain for more child-friendly roles or even start their own businesses. Equally, some fathers decide to become stay-at-home dads, to retrain or to go part-time.

Whatever you choose, try not to allow scare stories or guilt get in the way. Don't trust the headlines – I've seen working mothers blamed for everything from youth crime to unemployment, and, equally, I've seen stay-at-home mothers blamed for providing a 'bad example' to their children. (Interestingly, however, I've never seen a piece blaming working or stay-at-home fathers.) Whatever you do, unfortunately, you're likely to find people who will tell you you're doing the wrong thing. Blame seems to be an inevitable part of motherhood, whatever you choose to do, so it's best to ignore completely those who seek to undermine your choices and do what's right for you and your family.

If you plan to go back to work:

- Make sure you know what your rights are. Under new UK legislation, every parent with a child under six years of age or a disabled child under 18 years of age has the right to have a request for flexible working considered by their employer. The definition of 'flexible' could include different working hours or reduced working hours, the right to work from home or job-sharing.
- Ensure that you have childcare that suits your job. Childminders tend to be more flexible than nurseries, which have very set hours. However, the disadvantage is that, if your childminder is ill or unable to work for some other reason, you don't have anything to fall back on. Take your time finding suitable childcare. Contact your local authority for lists of approved, Ofsted-registered childminders and details of local nurseries. You can find au pairs and full-time and part-time nannies through local agencies – nanny shares with friends are also popular. All of these providers should be happy to meet you and your child as many times as you like and answer any questions you have. Trust your instincts when it comes to childcare – if something doesn't feel right, it probably isn't.
- Get organized. Juggling work and children is a challenge but it's not impossible. Decide with your partner who's going to do what chores around the home and who's going to do the picking up and dropping off. Get used to making up lunches and bags the night before to avoid frantic running around in the morning. And investigate small but crucial time-savers like internet shopping.

Joanne

I wanted to do something more meaningful, which was part of the reason why I retrained as a coach. I do measure work in terms of time away from my children and am much more choosy in terms of the things I say yes to. I have done all sorts of interesting jobs and met many interesting people, yet the only thing I've ever done which my kids are impressed with is work as a shop assistant in the Disney Store.

If you plan to stay at home:

- Decide with your partner who is going to be responsible for what. It may be that you're happy to take on more of the chores and the family 'administration' if you're staying at home; however, looking after a baby, especially in the first year, can be an all-consuming task. Feeling as if you're taking on too much can lead to feelings of resentment, so make sure you're happy with what you decide.
- Work on building your social networks, as discussed earlier in this chapter. It's important to have plenty of things you can do with your baby to avoid feeling isolated.
- Create a routine for yourself and your baby. This is particularly helpful in those early months when it seems as if you're doing nothing but feeding and changing. It could be something as simple as making sure you get out of the house every day in the afternoon, or signing up for classes, or having a regular afternoon at a friend's house.
- Make sure you don't neglect the things you enjoy doing. Staying at home doesn't mean looking after your child 24 hours a day, seven days a week, 365 days a year. Allow yourself to have some time off – you're doing a full-time job and you need time to yourself just like any other worker.

Be proud of yourself

It takes time to grow into your new role as a mother. However you choose to handle the future with your child, be sure in the knowledge that whatever you're doing is right. It must be, because it feels right for you and your family. Respect yourself and your new role.

Someone once asked me if I'd lost my identity after having my son. My response was no, I didn't lose my identity. I put it away in the back of my wardrobe. Sometimes I like to get it out and look at it every now and again. But the new one suits me pretty well.

Lucy

It's really important to me to be a good mother. I want our daughter to be able to look back at her childhood and remember it as a happy time. Without a doubt, that is the most important thing to me in my life right now. Prior to giving birth, I could think only about the sacrifices that would have to be made to accommodate a child. Now my thoughts are focused on providing a home for her where she knows she will always be loved, cared for and respected by us.

Afterword: Going forward

Recovering from PTSD or PND is a long road. Travelling that road could mean counselling, antidepressants or both. It may be that you'll have to take diversions along pathways that you never even knew existed or that you had long since erased from your mental map. Now that you've read this book, I hope that you'll feel less alone in your journey. Being convinced that you're the only person in the world who's ever had negative feelings connected with motherhood is very common. It helps so much when you know that many other people felt and still feel the same way as you.

It may not seem like it now, but life will return to normal – as normal as it can ever be with a new little person in your life. If you find the help you need, whatever it might be, you can start to enjoy your baby and your new family life. You will come to terms with what happened to you. That doesn't mean forgetting about it and trying to pretend it didn't happen. Those experiences are part of your life now, but they don't have to rule your life. It is possible to look back and say, 'Yes, that was awful, but I can deal with it now. I can move on.'

For some of us, moving on means having another baby. Others decide that their family is complete at one child. Whatever you decide, remember that, although having PND once makes it more likely you'll have it again, it's not a given and you will be a lot more prepared the second time a round.

Wherever your journey takes you, whatever you discover along the way, whatever joys and sadnesses accompany you, I hope this book has helped. It's a hard journey but the rewards are massive. You're doing a brilliant job. You are a mother. Therefore you are amazing. Good luck.

Joanne

Some people have more respect for me because they can see that I'm doing a hard job well. Also, becoming a mother has made me a better person, and I think this affects how others perceive me. I don't know though – ultimately I'm not at all bothered by what other people think of me. That's another gift my children have given me – the courage to be true to myself and not to give a toss about what the rest of the world thinks.

Useful contacts

Note that I have not included details of individual therapists or coaches. The websites of organizations such as the British Association for Counselling and Psychotherapy and the British Psychological Society provide the facility to search for a registered practitioner, and they also provide information on how to find a therapist. I strongly recommend that you go through these channels to find the right therapist for you.

Association for Improvements in the Maternity Services (AIMS)
1 Carlton Close
Camberley
Surrey GU15 1DS

Tel.: 0300 365 0663
Website: www.aims.org.uk
Advice: helpline@aims.org.uk
Website (Ireland): www.aimsireland.com
Advice (Ireland): info@aimsireland.com
AIMS is an organization that campaigns for better birth choices. The *AIMS Journal* is a great source of information on maternity issues.

Association for Post-Natal Illness (APNI)
145 Dawes Road
Fulham
London SW6 7EB

Helpline: 020 7386 0868 (10 a.m. to 2 p.m., Monday–Friday)
Website: https://apni.org (includes an online chat box)
A registered charity, APNI provides information leaflets, both for those experiencing postnatal illness and for healthcare professionals. It has a network of volunteers (telephone and postal) who have experienced postnatal illness themselves. The site is affiliated to <www.pni.org.uk>.

Australasian Birth Trauma Association (ABTA)
PO Box 3250
Norman Park QLD 4170

Tel.: 0412 445 770
Website: www.birthtrauma.org.au
Advice: Support@birthtrauma.org.au
This Australian charity was established in 2016 to support women and their families who are suffering postnatally from physical and/or psychological

trauma resulting from the birth process. It also offers education and support for health professionals who work with pre- and postnatal women.

Birthrights
Website: www.birthrights.org.uk
Advice: advice@birthrights.org.uk
Twitter: @birthrightsorg
Birthrights is the UK's only organization dedicated to improving women's experience of pregnancy and childbirth by promoting respect for human rights.

The Birth Trauma Association (BTA)
Email: support@birthtraumaassociation.org.uk
Website: https://birthtraumaassociation.org.uk
The BTA supports all women who have had a traumatic birth experience. The website contains birth stories, information on birth trauma, a reading list and details of counsellors who specialize in birth trauma.

The British Association for Counselling and Psychotherapy (BACP)
15 St John's Business Park
Lutterworth
Leicestershire LE17 4HB

Tel.: 01455 883300
Website: www.bacp.co.uk
The BACP is a professional body for counsellors and psychotherapists in the UK. You can search their database of registered therapists by area and specialist subject – read their section on 'Finding the right therapist' for information on how to find an accredited practitioner who's right for you.

The British Psychological Society (BPS)
St Andrew's House
48 Princess Road East
Leicester LE1 7DR

Tel.: 0116 254 9568
Website: www.bps.org.uk
You can use its 'Find a psychologist' pages on the website to find practitioners who specialize in PTSD or PND in your area, and also to check that they are registered.

EMDR Association UK & Ireland
PO Box 3356
Swindon
SN2 9EE

Website: https://emdrassociation.org.uk
Enquiries: info@emdrassociation.org.uk
The website includes a searchable directory of accredited therapists.

Fathers Reaching Out
Website: www.reachingoutpmh.co.uk
Email: info@reachingoutpmh.co.uk
Twitter: @markwilliamsFMH
Founder Mark Williams campaigns for better support for fathers' mental health.

The Lullaby Trust
Audley House
13 Palace Street
London SW1E 5HX

Website: www.lullabytrust.org.uk
Support: 0808 802 6868
Information and advice: 0808 802 6869
The site also provides safer sleeping guidelines for you and your baby.

Mind
Mind (England):
15–19 Broadway
Stratford
London E15 4BQ

Mind Cymru:
3rd Floor, Castlebridge 4, Castlebridge
5–19 Cowbridge Road East
Cardiff CF11 9AB

Website: www.mind.org.uk
MindinfoLine (advice line): 0300 123 3393
Mind is England's and Wales's leading mental-health charity, which exists to help anyone with any kind of mental illness, including PND. It produces a range of booklets, including one on PND, and the advice line is staffed by specialists.

The Scottish Association for Mental Health
Brunswick House
51 Wilson Street
Glasgow, G1 1UZ

Website: www.samh.org.uk
SAMH is Scotland's leading mental-health charity, which exists to help anyone with any kind of mental illness, including PND.

Inspire
Central Office
Lombard House
10–20 Lombard Street
Belfast BT1 1RD

Website: www.inspirewellbeing.org
Inspire is Northern Ireland's leading mental-health and wellbeing charity, which exists to help anyone with any kind of mental illness, including PND.

Mumsnet
Website: www.mumsnet.com
A website used by thousands of parents with conversations covering everything from nappy rash to education policies, Mumsnet can be a fantastic source of support for those with birth trauma or PND and those having trouble adjusting to parenthood. Comments are largely unmoderated, so bear in mind that you may not always get the responses you're looking for, but generally the community is extremely supportive and welcoming. (However, it's a good idea to steer clear of the 'Am I being unreasonable?' forum if you're feeling vulnerable, as the debate on this particular forum can be pretty robust.)

Netmums
Website: www.netmums.com
Another board used by thousands of parents, Netmums is more heavily moderated than Mumsnet but, again, the range of conversations is vast and the community extremely supportive. Netmums also has a special area where mothers can organize meet-ups.

Family Lives
15–17 The Broadway
Hatfield
Hertfordshire AL9 5HZ

Helpline: 0808 800 2222
Website: www.familylives.org.uk
Family Lives is a national charity dedicated to helping mothers and fathers in all aspects of parenting. The website has lots of useful information and advice.

PATTCh
http://pattch.org
This US charity aims to expand awareness and advance knowledge about traumatic birth and its adverse impact on babies and childbearing people.

Post Natal Illness
Website: www.pni.org.uk
This information website is run by those affected by postnatal illness and those who have come through it, for others in the same situation.

Relate
Website: www.relate.org.uk
Relate offers advice, relationship counselling, sex therapy, workshops, mediation, consultations and support face to face, by phone and through its website. You can find your nearest branch and its contact details on the website, plus details of Relate publications.

Samaritans
Helpline (24 hours): 116 123 (including the Republic of Ireland)
Website: www.samaritans.org
Email: jo@samaritans.org
The Samaritans provide confidential emotional support 24 hours a day to those experiencing despair, distress or suicidal feelings.

Trauma and Birth Stress (TABS)
PO Box 18002
Glen Innes
Auckland
New Zealand

Website: www.tabs.org.nz
This organization's website has a wealth of information about PTSD, including up-to-date research and parents' stories. It's also a point of contact for professionals wishing to find people who might be willing to share their experiences for research purposes.

Twins and Multiple Births Association (TAMBA)
Manor House
Church Hill
Aldershot
Hampshire GU12 4JU

Advice line: 0800 138 0509 (daily 10 a.m. to 1 p.m. and 7 p.m. to 10 p.m.)
Website: www.tamba.org.uk
This is a great resource for parents of twins or more, providing information and support networks.

References

1 Coming to terms with a traumatic birth

Adewuya, A. O., Ologu, Y. A. and Ibigbami, O. S., 'Post-traumatic stress disorder after childbirth in Nigerian women: prevalence and risk factors', *British Journal of Obstetrics and Gynaecology*, vol. 113 (2006), pp. 284–8.

'Administration of chloroform to Queen Victoria' [editorial], *The Lancet*, vol. 1 (1853), p. 452.

Allen, S., 'A qualitative analysis of the process, mediating variables and impact of traumatic childbirth', *Journal of Reproductive and Infant Psychology*, vol. 16 (1998), pp. 107–31.

American Psychiatric Association, Diagnostic and Statistical Manual of Mental Disorders (DSM III). American Psychiatric Association, Washington, DC, 1980.

American Psychiatric Association, Diagnostic and Statistical Manual of Mental Disorders, Fourth Edition, Text Revision (DSM-IV-TR). American Psychiatric Association, Washington, DC, 2000.

American Psychiatric Association factsheet on PTSD DSM 5 available from <https://www.psychiatry.org/psychiatrists/practice/dsm/educational -resources/dsm-5-fact-sheets>

Antenatal and Postnatal Mental Health Guidelines: Clinical Management and Service Guidelines. NICE clinical guideline no. 45. National Institute for Health and Clinical Excellence, London, 2007,<https://www.nice.org. uk/guidance/cg192/evidence/full-guideline-pdf-4840896925>.

Ayers, Susan, Wright, Daniel B. and Thornton, Alexandra, 'Development of a measure of postpartum PTSD: The City Birth Trauma Scale', *Frontiers in Psychiatry*, vol. 9 (2018); available online: <https://www. frontiersin.org/articles/10.3389/fpsyt.2018.00409/full>

Beck, Cheryl Tatano, 'Birth trauma: in the eye of the beholder', *Nursing Research*, vol. 53 (2004), pp. 28–35.

Beck, Cheryl Tatano, 'Post-traumatic stress disorder due to childbirth: the aftermath', *Nursing Research*, vol. 53 (2004), pp. 216–24.

Creedy, Debra K., Shochet, Ian M. and Horsfall, Jan, 'Childbirth and the development of acute trauma symptoms: incidence and contributing factors', *Birth*, vol. 27 (2000), pp. 104–11.

Crompton, Judy, 'Post-traumatic stress disorder and childbirth', Auckland, New Zealand, 2000, <www.tabs.org.nz/pdfdocs/jrcrompton%20tabs.pdf>.

Czarnocka, J. and Slade, P., 'Prevalence and predictors of post-traumatic stress symptoms following childbirth', *British Journal of Clinical Psychology*, vol. 39 (2000), pp. 35–51.

Dick-Read, Grantly, *Childbirth without Fear: The Principles and Practice of Natural Childbirth*, 2nd edn. Pinter & Martin, London, 2007.

Ellis, Richard H., ed., 'The case books of Dr John Snow', *Medical History Supplement*, No. 14 (1994), p. 271.

Gamble, Jenny, Creedy, Debra, Moyle, Wendy, Webster, Joan, McAllister, Margaret and Dickson, Paul, 'Effectiveness of a counseling intervention after a traumatic childbirth: a randomized controlled trial', *Birth*, vol. 32 (2005), pp. 11–19.

Lally, Joanne E., Murtagh, Madeleine J., Macphail, Sheila and Thomson, Richard G., 'More in hope than expectation: women's experience and expectations of pain relief in labour: a review', *BMC Medicine*, vol. 6 (2008), p. 7.

Söderquist J., Wijma K. and Wijma B., 'Traumatic stress after childbirth: the role of obstetric variables', *Journal of Psychosomatic Obstetrics and Gynaecology*, vol. 23 (2002), pp. 31–9.

Soet, Johanna E., Brack, Gregory A. and DiIorio, Colleen, 'Prevalence and predictors of women's experience of psychological trauma during childbirth', *Birth*, vol. 30 (2003), pp. 36–46.

Yildiz, PD., Ayers, S., Phillips, L., 'The prevalence of posttraumatic stress disorder in pregnancy and after birth: a systematic review and meta-analysis', *Journal of Affective Disorders*, vol. 221 (2017), pp. 238–245.

2 Postnatal depression and puerperal psychosis

4 Child survey <https://www.nhs.uk/news/pregnancy-and-child/postnatal-depression-often-unreported/>

American Psychiatric Association, Diagnostic and Statistical Manual of Mental Disorders, Fourth Edition, Text Revision (DSM-IV-TR). American Psychiatric Association, Washington, DC, 2000.

Antenatal and Postnatal Mental Health Guidelines: Clinical Management and Service Guidelines. NICE clinical guideline no. 45. National Institute for Health and Clinical Excellence, London, 2007, <www.nice.org.uk/nice media/pdf/CG045NICEGuidelineCorrected.pdf>.

Appleby L., Warner R., Whitton A. and Faragher, B., 'A controlled study of fluoxetine and cognitive-behavioural counselling in the treatment of postnatal depression', *BMJ*, vol. 314 (1997), pp. 932–6.

Beck, Cheryl Tatano, 'Postpartum depression: a metasynthesis', *Qualitative Health Research*, vol. 12 (2002), p. 453.

Boath, E., Bradley, E. and Henshaw, C., 'Women's views of antidepressants in the treatment of postnatal depression', *Journal of Psychosomatic Obstetrics and Gynaecology*, vol. 25 (2004), pp. 221–33.

Brimelow, Adam, 'Health visitor numbers "falling"', BBC Online, 23 February 2007, <news.bbc.co.uk/1/hi/health/6388397.stm>.

Dennis, C. L., Ross, L. E. and Herxheimer, A., 'Oestrogens and progestins for preventing and treating postpartum depression', *Cochrane Database of Systematic Reviews 1999*, Issue 3, Art. no. CD001690, <www.cochrane.org/reviews/en/ab001690.html>.

Halbreich, Uriel and Karkun, Sandhya, 'Cross-cultural and social diversity of prevalence of postpartum depression and depressive symptoms', *Journal of Affective Disorders*, vol. 91 (2006), pp. 97–111.

Hall, P. L. and Wittkowski, A., 'An exploration of negative thoughts as a normal phenomenon after childbirth', *Journal of Midwifery and Women's Health*, vol. 51 (2006), pp. 321–30.

Hay, D. F. and Pawlby S., 'Prosocial development in relation to children's and mothers' psychological problems', *Child Development*, vol. 74 (2003), pp. 1314–27.

Hipwell, A. E., Murray, L., Ducournau, P. and Stein, A., 'The effects of maternal depression and parental conflict on children's peer play', *Child: Care, Health and Development*, vol. 31 (2005), pp. 11–23.

Kurstjens, Sophie and Wolke, Dieter, 'Effects of maternal depression on cognitive development of children over the first 7 years of life', *Journal of Child Psychology and Psychiatry*, vol. 42 (2001), pp. 623–36.

Milgrom, Jeannette, Negri, Lisa M., Gemmill, Alan W., McNeil, Margaret and Martin, Paul R., 'A randomized controlled trial of psychological interventions for postnatal depression', *British Journal of Clinical Psychology*, vol. 44 (2005), pp. 529–42.

Milgrom, Jeannette, Westley, Doreen T. and Gemmill, Alan W., 'The mediating role of maternal responsiveness in some longer term effects of postnatal depression on infant development', *Infant Behavior and Development*, vol. 27 (2004), pp. 443–54.

Misri, S., Reebye, P., Corral, M. and Mills, L., 'The use of paroxetine and cognitive-behavioural therapy in postpartum depression and anxiety: a randomized controlled trial', *Journal of Clinical Psychiatry*, vol. 65 (2004), pp. 1236–41.

O'Hara, M. W., Stuart, S., Gorman, L. L. and Wenzel, A., 'Efficacy of interpersonal psychotherapy for postpartum depression', *Archives of General Psychiatry*, vol. 57 (2000), pp. 1039–45.

'Postnatal depression soars, say midwives', press release from the Royal College of Midwifery, 30 April 2007, <https://www.who.int/mental_health/maternal-child/maternal_mental_health/en/>.

Reissland, Nadja, Hopkins, Brian, Helms, Peter and Williams, Bob, 'Maternal stress and depression and the lateralisation of infant cradling', *Journal of Child Psychology and Psychiatry*, 2007, <doi:10.1111/j.1469-7610.2007.01791.x>.

Robertson, Emma and Lyons, Antonia, 'Living with puerperal psychosis: a qualitative analysis', *Psychology and Psychotherapy: Theory, Research and Practice*, vol. 76 (2003), pp. 411–31.

Triggle, Nick, 'Postnatal mental care "lacking"', BBC Online, 18 April 2007, <news.bbc.co.uk/1/hi/health/6564293.stm>.

Wisner, Katherine L., Perel, James M., Peindl, Kathleen S., Hanusa, Barbara H., Findling, Robert L. and Rapport, D. J., 'Prevention of recurrent postpartum depression: a randomized clinical trial', *Journal of Clinical Psychiatry*, vol. 62 (2001), pp. 82–8.

Wisner, Katherine L., Perel, James M., Peindl, Kathleen S., Hanusa, Barbara H., Piontek, Catherine M. and Findling, Robert L., 'Prevention of postpartum depression: a pilot randomized clinical trial', *American Journal of Psychiatry*, vol. 161 (2004), pp. 1290–2.

World Health Organization, *International Statistical Classification of Diseases and Related Health Problems*, 10th Revision. Version for 2007. World Health Organization, Geneva, 2007, <www.who.int/classifications/apps/icd/icd10online/>.

'Written evidence from the Institute of Health Visiting to the parliamentary Health and Social Care Committee inquiry into the First 1000 Days of Life', report from Institute of Health Visiting, 6 September 2018, <https://ihv.org.uk/news-and-views/news/ihv-publishes-submission-to-parliamentary-inquiry-into-the-first-1000-days-of-life/>.

3 Learning to love your baby

Ainsworth, M., *Deprivation of Maternal Care: A Reassessment of its Effects*. World Health Organization, Geneva, 1962.

Bellieni, C. V., Ceccarelli, D., Rossi, F., Buonocore, G., Maffei, M., Perrone, S. and Petraglia, F., 'Is prenatal bonding enhanced by prenatal education courses?' *Minerva Ginecologica*, vol. 59 (2007), pp. 125–9.

Bowlby, J., *Maternal Care and Mental Health*. World Health Organization, Geneva, 1951.

Feldman, R., Weller, A., Zagoory-Sharon, O. and Levine, A., 'Level of oxytocin in pregnant women predicts mother–child bond', *Psychological Science*, vol. 18 (2007), pp. 965–70.

Klier, C. M., 'Mother–infant bonding disorders in patients with postnatal depression: The Postpartum Bonding Questionnaire in clinical practice', *Archives of Women's Mental Health*, vol. 9 (2006), pp. 289–91.

Kumar, R. C., '"Anybody's child": severe disorders of mother-to-infant bonding', *British Journal of Psychiatry*, vol. 171 (1997), pp. 175–81.

Moehler, E., Brunner, R., Wiebel, A., Reck, C. and Resch, F., 'Maternal depressive symptoms in the postnatal period are associated with long-term impairment of mother–child bonding', *Archives of Women's Mental Health*, vol. 9 (2006), pp. 273–8.

Righetti-Veltema, M., Bousquet, A. and Manzano, J., 'Impact of postpartum depressive symptoms on mother and her 18-month-old infant', *European Child and Adolescent Psychiatry*, vol. 12 (2003), pp. 75–83.

Rutter, Michael, 'Nature, nurture, and development: from evangelism through science toward policy and practice', *Child Development*, vol. 73 (2002), pp. 1–21.

Sluckin, A., '"My baby doesn't need me": understanding bonding failure', *Health Visitor*, vol. 66, pp. 409–12 (1993), 414.

Stern, N. B., 'Motherhood: the emotional awakening', *Journal of Pediatric Health Care*, vol. 13 (1999), pp. S8–12.

4 Family affairs

DiLillo, D. and Damashek, A., 'Parenting characteristics of women reporting a history of childhood sexual abuse', *Child Maltreatment*, vol. 8 (2003), pp. 319–33.

Doyle, Celia, 'Surviving and coping with emotional abuse in childhood', *Clinical Child Psychology and Psychiatry*, vol. 6 (2001), pp. 387–402.

Schuetze, P. and Eiden, R. D., 'The relationship between sexual abuse during childhood and parenting outcomes: modeling direct and indirect pathways', *Child Abuse and Neglect*, vol. 29 (2005), pp. 645–59.

Susin, L. R., Giugliani, E. R. and Kummer, S. C., 'Influence of grandmothers on breastfeeding practices', *Revista de Saúde Pública*, vol. 39 (2005), pp. 141–7.

5 Baby makes three: your new relationship with your partner

Alder, E. M., 'Sexual behaviour in pregnancy, after childbirth and during breast-feeding', *Baillières Clinical Obstetrics and Gynaecology*, vol. 3 (1989), pp. 805–21.

Barrett, G., Pendry, E., Peacock, J., Victor, C., Thakar, R. and Manyonda, I., 'Women's sexuality after childbirth: a pilot study', *Archives of Sexual Behavior*, vol. 28 (1999), pp. 179–91.

Barrett, G., Pendry, E., Peacock, J., Victor, C., Thakar, R. and Manyonda, I., 'Women's sexual health after childbirth', *British Journal of Obstetrics and Gynaecology*, vol. 107 (2000), pp. 186–95.

Davidson, Clare, 'Single women "do less housework"', BBC Online, 23 February 2007, <https://news.bbc.co.uk/1/hi/business/6382429.stm>.

Fägerskiöld, A., 'A change in life as experienced by first-time fathers', *Scandinavian Journal of Caring Sciences*, vol. 22 (2008), pp. 64–71.

Goldberg, W. A., Michaels, G. Y. and Lamb, M. E., 'Husbands' and wives' adjustment to pregnancy and first parenthood', *Journal of Family Issues*, vol. 6 (1985), pp. 483–503.

Henwood, K. and Procter, J., 'The "good father": reading men's accounts of paternal involvement during the transition to first-time fatherhood', *Social Psychology*, vol. 42 (2003), pp. 337–55.

Kluwer, Esther S. and Johnson, Matthew D., 'Conflict frequency and relationship quality across the transition to parenthood', *Journal of Marriage and Family*, vol. 69 (2007), p. 1089.

Lawrence, Erika, Rothman, Alexia D., Cobb, Rebecca J., Rothman, Michael T. and Bradbury, Thomas N., 'Marital satisfaction across the transition to parenthood', *Journal of Family Psychology*, vol. 22 (2008), pp. 41–50.

Morof, D., Barrett, G., Peacock, J., Victor, C. R. and Manyonda, I., 'Postnatal depression and sexual health after childbirth', *Obstetrics and Gynaecology*, vol. 102 (2003), pp. 1318–25.

Olin, R. M. and Faxelid, E., 'Parents' needs to talk about their experiences of childbirth', *Scandinavian Journal of Caring Sciences*, vol. 17 (2003), pp. 153–9.

O'Malley, D., Higgins, A., Begley, C., Daly, D. and Smith, V., 'Prevalence of and risk factors associated with sexual health issues in primiparous women at 6 and 12 months postpartum; a longitudinal prospective cohort study (the MAMMI study)', *BMC Pregnancy and Childbirth*, vol. 18 (2018), <https://bmcpregnancychildbirth.biomedcentral.com/articles/10.1186/s12884-018-1838-6>.

Paulson, James L, Dauber, Sarah, and Leiferman, Jenn A. 'Individual and Combined Effects of Postpartum Depression in Mothers and Fathers on Parenting Behavior', *Pediatrics*, vol. 118, issue 2 (2006), pp. 659–68.

Pastore, L., Owens, A. and Raymond, C., 'Postpartum sexuality concerns among first-time parents from one U.S. academic hospital', *Journal of Sexual Medicine*, vol. 4 (2007), pp. 115–23.

Premberg, A., Hellström, A. L. and Berg, M., 'Experiences of the first year as father', *Scandinavian Journal of Caring Sciences*, vol. 22 (2008), pp. 56–63.

Rowland, M., Foxcroft, L., Hopman, W. M. and Patel, R., 'Breastfeeding and sexuality immediately post partum', *Canadian Family Physician*, vol. 51 (2005), pp. 1366–7.

Shapiro, A. F., Gottman, J. M. and Carrère, S., 'The baby and the marriage: identifying factors that buffer against decline in marital satisfaction after the first baby arrives', *Journal of Family Psychology*, vol. 14 (2000), pp. 59–70.

Woranitat, W. and Taneepanichskul, S., 'Sexual function during the postpartum period', *Journal of the Medical Association of Thailand*, vol. 90 (2007), pp. 1744–8.

6 Adjusting to a new you

Amorim, A. R., Linne, Y. M. and Lourenco, P. M., 'Diet or exercise, or both, for weight reduction in women carrying excess weight after childbirth', *Cochrane Database of Systematic Reviews 2007*, Issue 3, Art. no. CD005627, <www.cochrane.org/reviews/en/ab005627.html>.

Berger, A., Peragallo-Urrutia, R. and Nicholson, W., 'Systematic review of the effect of individual and combined nutrition and exercise interventions on weight, adiposity and metabolic outcomes after delivery: evidence for developing behavioural guidelines for post-partum weight control', *BMC Pregnancy and Childbirth*, vol. 14 (2014), <https://www.ncbi.nlm.nih.gov/pubmed/25208549>.

'New mums feel pressure to be slim', BBC Online, 3 February 2005, <https://news.bbc.co.uk/1/hi/health/4232009.stm>.

Orbach, S. and Rubin, H., 'Two for the price of one: the impact of body image during pregnancy and after birth', Government Equalities Office, 2014, <https://www.gov.uk/government/publications/two-for-the-price-of-one>.

Rallis, S., Skouteris, H., Wertheim, E. H. and Paxton, S. J., 'Predictors of body image during the first year postpartum: a prospective study', *Women's Health*, vol. 45 (2007), pp. 87–104.

Further reading

Bruijn, Melissa and Gould, Debby, *How to Heal a Bad Birth: Making Sense, Making Peace and Moving On*. Birthtalk.org, 2017 [ebook only]. A gentle guide for women who have experienced a difficult, disappointing or traumatic birth.

Cusk, Rachel, *A Life's Work: On Becoming a Mother*. Fourth Estate, London, 2001. Meditations on the darker side of motherhood.

Figes, Kate and Zimmerman, Jean, *Life after Birth: What Even Your Friends Won't Tell You about Motherhood*. St Martin's Press, Basingstoke, 2001. Dispelling the myths surrounding modern motherhood.

Kitzinger, Sheila, *Birth Crisis*. Routledge, Oxford, 2006. An analysis of the way we give birth today and what's gone wrong for many mothers. Aimed at both professionals and lay people.

Stadlen, Naomi, *What Mothers Do: Especially When It Looks Like Nothing*. Piatkus, London, 2005. A real confidence booster if you feel you're not getting anywhere with your baby.

Thomas, Kim, *Birth Trauma: A Guide for You, Your Friends and Family to Coping with Post-Traumatic Stress Disorder Following Birth*. Nell James Publishers, 2013. Everything you and your family and friends need to know about birth trauma: what causes it, how it affects your personal relationships, how to treat it and where to find support.

Williams, Mark, *Daddy Blues: Postnatal Depression and Fatherhood*. Trigger, Newark, Nottinghamshire, 2018. A first-hand account of a father's mental health struggles.

Index